To our partners who tolerate our absence on frequent tours of duty

The royalties of this book are donated to the Army Benevolent Fund

TRAUMA RULES 2

INCORPORATING
MILITARY TRAUMA RULES

COLONEL
Tim Hodgetts

QHP OStJ MMEd FRCP FRCSEd FFAEM FIMCRCSEd FRGS L/RAMC
Honorary Professor of Emergency Medicine and Trauma, University of Birmingham, UK;
Defence Consultant Adviser in Emergency Medicine, Royal Centre for Defence Medicine

AND

MAJOR
Lee Turner

RN BSc(Hons) RNZNC
Officer Commanding 2nd Health Support Team
Palmerston North, New Zealand

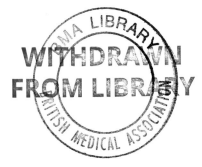

Blackwell
Publishing

BMJ
Books

© 1997 BMJ Publishing Group
© 2006 Tim Hodgetts and Lee Turner
Published by Blackwell Publishing Ltd
BMJ Books is an imprint of the BMJ Publishing Group Limited, used under licence

Blackwell Publishing, Inc., 350 Main Street, Malden, Massachusetts 02148-5020, USA
Blackwell Publishing Ltd, 9600 Garsington Road, Oxford OX4 2DQ, UK
Blackwell Publishing Asia Pty Ltd, 550 Swanston Street, Carlton, Victoria 3053, Australia

The right of the Author to be identified as the Author of this Work has been asserted in accordance with the Copyright, Designs and Patents Act 1988.

First published 1997
Second edition 2006

1 2006

Library of Congress Cataloging-in-Publication Data

Hodgetts, T. J.
    Trauma rules 2 : incorporating military trauma rules / Tim Hodgetts,
Lee Turner.
        p. ; cm.
    Rev. ed. of: Trauma rules. 1997.
    Includes index.
    ISBN-13: 978-0-7279-1649-5 (alk. paper)
    ISBN-10: 0-7279-1649-1 (alk. paper)
    1. Wounds and injuries—Treatment—Handbooks, manuals, etc.
    2. Critical care medicine—Handbooks, manuals, etc.   3. Intensive care
units—Handbooks, manuals, etc.   I. Turner, Lee, 1966– .
    II. Hodgetts, T. J. Trauma rules.   III. Title.   IV. Title: Trauma rules
two.
    [DNLM: 1. Emergencies—Handbooks.   2. Emergency Medicine
—methods—Handbooks.   3. Wounds and Injuries—Handbooks.
WB 39 H689t 2006]
RD93.H63 2006
617.1—dc22
                                                                2006019245

ISBN-13: 978-0-7279-1649-5
ISBN-10: 0-7279-1649-1

A catalogue record for this title is available from the British Library

Set in 8.75/11pt Palatino by Graphicraft Limited, Hong Kong
Printed and bound in India by Replika Press Pvt., Ltd

Commissioning Editor: Mary Banks
Development Editor: Julie Elliott
Production Controller: Debbie Wyer

For further information on Blackwell Publishing, visit our website:
http://www.blackwellpublishing.com

Contents

CONTENTS

Investigation and definitive care

Contributors

Second edition

Lieutenant Colonel Peter Mahoney OStJ TD RAMC
Senior Lecturer in Critical Care, Royal Centre for Defence Medicine
Lieutenant Colonel Malcolm Russell RAMC
Senior Lecturer in Pre-hospital Emergency Medicine, Royal Centre for Defence Medicine
Captain Simon Davies OStJ QARANC(V)
Trauma Research Nurse, Royal Centre for Defence Medicine
Leading Naval Nurse Claire Snead QARNNS
Project Officer, Royal Centre for Defence Medicine

First edition

Professor Stephen Deane
Professor of Surgery, Liverpool, New South Wales, Australia
Keith Gunning
General and Trauma Surgeon, Newcastle, UK
Professor Ken Hillman
Intensive Care Specialist, Liverpool, New South Wales, Australia
Stuart Matthews
Orthopaedic and Trauma Surgeon, Leeds, UK
Professor Peter Roberts
Surgeon, Royal Army Medical Corps, UK
Maria Seger
Trauma Nurse Consultant, Liverpool, New South Wales, Australia
Michael Sugrue
Surgeon, Director of Trauma, Liverpool, New South Wales, Australia

Preface to the second edition

This second edition of *Trauma Rules* has been expanded (there are 14 new rules) and thoroughly updated to take account of changes in trauma care practice in the last decade. You will find that many of the rules have multiple references that give weight to your teaching or directions in the resuscitation room.

Perhaps the greatest change in this edition is the addition of military trauma rules. Military trauma is different. There is a different pattern of injury to civilian practice, different human resources and limited diagnostic and treatment facilities in the field. Where important differences exist these are highlighted. But military trauma care is not necessarily to a lesser standard. Indeed, by reading the military rules you will learn a new paradigm for trauma care and be exposed to cutting edge practices that may not yet be widely exploited in civilian trauma care.

We are sure you will enjoy this second edition: above all, learning must be fun!

Tim Hodgetts
Lee Turner
Birmingham and Palmerston North
2006

Preface to the first edition

The management of major trauma may seem to be a complex issue but it can be approached in a systematic manner. This book combines a systematic approach with a novel series of trauma rules to trigger the memory when faced with a seriously injured patient.

Each rule is accompanied by the reason, the exceptions to the rule and, where appropriate, an illustration highlighting a key aspect of the rule.

Learning should be fun, and this book is designed to be fun to read. It is hoped that these trauma rules may be used by those involved in trauma education at all professional levels to emphasize the key issues in trauma management and to perpetuate a high standard of trauma care.

Trauma Rules is an *aide memoire* and supplements existing textbooks on this subject. Readers who require a more extensive understanding of the management of trauma are referred to the following books, also published by BMJ Publishing Group.

- *ABC of Major Trauma*
- *Trauma: Beyond the Resuscitation Room*

Tim Hodgetts
Stephen Deane
Keith Gunning
London and Sydney

Rules are made to be broken,
That's not what you should do.
For one of these days these rules
Will help you save a life or two.

The primary directives

Anxiety provokes memory loss: so learn a system and stick to it

The reason

When the chips are down you may only have your own experience to rely on. When your experience is limited you need rules that are easy to remember and easy to apply, even in the most threatening of circumstances. This system is:

Airway, with control of the cervical spine;
Breathing, with oxygen; and
Circulation, with control of external blood loss.

This **ABC** system allows the identification and treatment of life-threatening injuries in a rapid, logical and reproducible order. The patient assessment is extended to include:

Disability (neurological status); and
Exposure, with environmental considerations (control of body temperature).

Together, the initial patient assessment following this **ABCDE** system is known as the 'primary survey'. This is the systematic approach taught on the internationally established *Advanced Trauma Life Support* course [1] (adapted as the *Early Management of Severe Trauma* course in Australia) and *Pre-hospital Trauma Life Support* course [2].

The exceptions

To the beginner in trauma management, there are no exceptions to this rule. This is your code of practice. The experienced clinician, however, will regard all rules as guidelines but will still closely follow **ABC** principles.

The most common cause of avoidable death in a military conflict is uncontrolled external haemorrhage, particularly from the limbs, following blast and penetrating trauma. Champion has demonstrated that 50% of US battlefield deaths in Vietnam were from exsanguination. Eighty per cent of these were torso injury and 20% were from *'injured vessels that might be controlled by pressure'* (neck, limbs, soft tissues) [3]. Military practice has therefore modified the ABC paradigm (within the *Battlefield Advanced Trauma Life Support* course [4]) to **<C>ABCDE**:

    <C> Control of catastrophic haemorrhage;
    A   Airway, with control of the cervical spine *where appropriate*;
    B   Breathing, with oxygen *where available*; and
    C   Circulation, with control of non-catastrophic external haemorrhage.

Spinal immobilization is designed to protect the cord following blunt trauma with hyperextension/hyperflexion that results in ligamentous instability: the cervical spine will not benefit from immobilization following penetrating trauma.

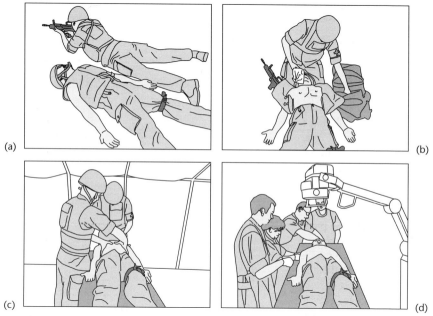

Figure 2.1 The stages of military resuscitation. (a) Care under fire. (b) Tactical field care. (c) Field resuscitation. (d) Advanced resuscitation.

All 4 one and one for all

The reason

Common principles can be applied to trauma resuscitation from point of wounding to casualty reception at hospital. In other words there is *one system for all* patients and all injury mechanisms. This is the **<C>ABC** system (see Rule 1).

The capability for trauma resuscitation increases incrementally along the chain of evacuation, with progressively more experienced clinical staff undertaking a greater scope of interventions, supported by a greater choice of diagnostic and treatment options.

In the military there are four clearly definable levels of clinical capability:

1 *Care under fire.* Care while the bullets are still flying is understandably limited and may include application of a tourniquet to arrest catastrophic haemorrhage (**<C>**) together with postural airway drainage (**A**)—lie the casualty face down, or preferably in the *recovery* or *three-quarters prone* position. This may be achievable by self-aid or require buddy aid (first aid).

2 *Tactical field care.* Care at point of wounding (including, for example, a vehicle entrapment) delivered by trained clinical personnel while recognizing a continuing potential security threat (the so-called 'semi-permissive environment').

3 *Field resuscitation.* Team-based trauma care far forward in a field environment, with the team led by a doctor trained in resuscitation principles and supported by paramedical +/− nursing staff. There would be no imaging capability, no surgical intervention and no blood available. This is the level of care referred to in the army as the Regimental Aid Post (RAP) or Battalion Aid Station.

4 *Advanced resuscitation.* Team-based trauma care led by a specialist (emergency physician) and involving, for example, a multidisciplinary team of an anaesthetist, surgeon and specialist emergency medicine nurses. There are diagnostic and interventional skills that are not available further forward.

The exceptions

The ubiquitous civilian trauma care paradigm currently remains as **ABC**. While there is a progressive capability from pre-hospital to hospital, this is defined by the training and equipment of the provider rather than constrained by the threat to physical security.

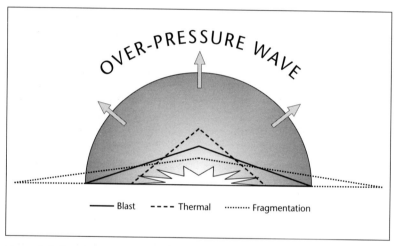

Figure 3.1 Blast injury patterns over distance.

Civilian and military trauma care is different

The reason

There are a number of features that differentiate trauma care in a military operational environment from that in a civilian environment.

Injury pattern. Military trauma generates injury patterns rarely seen in civilian practice, with multiple fragment wounds, blast injury to the lung and bowel, avulsive amputations and contaminated ballistic wounds.

Population at risk. A military population is predominantly males aged 18–40 who have a low co-morbidity for chronic conditions. Children, the elderly and pregnant females will be encountered when the local population is eligible for treatment (and international humanitarian law demands that any individual will be offered *emergency life-saving treatment* who presents to the military medical services).

Physical factors. There may be an adverse climate, with limited climate control; power is unreliable and procedures may have to be undertaken in minimal lighting conditions and without power-dependent diagnostic imaging (plain radiography; computed tomography [CT]); there may be no running water for optimal hygiene; tented treatment areas are difficult to keep clean (for example, high dust level in desert).

Security. Staff may be working under threat of ballistic, blast or chemical attack. Combat body armour and helmets may need to be worn while attending casualties, even in a hospital setting.

Equipment and drugs. You have what you have. The supply chain may be many thousands of miles long and if the resupply chain is interrupted there is no option other than to improvise or make do. Traditionally, diagnostic equipment is reduced compared to civilian best practice: there may be no diagnostic ultrasound, no CT and no angiography. Interventional radiologists will not be deployed with the small field hospital units.

People. The Trauma Team in a UK field hospital is based on consultants (specialists) in all relevant disciplines who are available 24 hours/day to receive the wounded. This model is reproduced in very few civilian centres in the UK. *Seniority saves time* in that decisions are made quickly regarding movement to the operating theatre and all critical procedures can be undertaken by senior staff (specifically, the presence of a trauma surgeon on the Trauma Team improves in-hospital trauma system function, although it has no measurable effect on patient outcome [5]). However, in a multiple casualty situation there are limited off-duty staff on whom to draw.

Continued

Focus. A field hospital is specifically configured for the reception and rapid surgical intervention for those injured in combat. This is its core business. Civilian hospitals will not universally share this same system configuration and preparedness to deal with major trauma (with the exception of designated major trauma centres).

The exceptions

Blunt trauma, particularly motor vehicle crashes, accounts for an increasing proportion of trauma in an enduring operation. The more enduring an operation becomes, the closer the diagnostic capabilities and treatment environment approximates to civilian standards. Military patterns of injury are increasingly seen in the civilian setting as a result of terrorist bombs.

Table 3.1 Explosive device.

Mechanism	Effects
Blast wave	The wave of over-pressure caused by compression of air by a rapidly expanding sphere of hot gas. Results in perforation of bowel, rupture of eardrum and intra-alveolar haemorrhage (*blast lung*)
Blast wind	Rush of air behind blast wind. Carries debris, resulting in fragmentation injury. Causes knock-down blunt trauma. Results in avulsive amputations
Fragmentation	The most frequent injury and commonly multiple wounds. Fragments from the device may be primary (the bomb case) or secondary (packed around the explosive, such as notched wire in a grenade or nails in improvised device)
Burns	Often superficial and confined to exposed areas; if close to explosion may be full thickness
Crush	Explosions in a confined space may result in crush. Blast wave is reinforced on reflection from walls and ceiling increasing the severity of blast injury
Psychological	The aim of a terrorist is to induce fear and change behaviour

Preparation

Any time preparing is time well spent *or* Prior Planning and Preparation Prevents Poor Performance

The reason

Time taken to prepare people, equipment, drugs and space will optimize the smooth running of the resuscitation when the patient arrives.

People. The Team Leader should assign roles to the assembling members of the Trauma Team and ensure each is wearing appropriate personal protective equipment (see Rule 6). Who is to manage the airway? Who will do the primary survey? Who will obtain intravenous access, take blood and send the samples to the laboratory? Who will cut off the clothes? Who will attach the monitors? Who will record all the clinical findings (the scribe)? Roles can be identified by tabards, which have increased value in a large hospital where on-duty specialist staff are not well known to each other.

Equipment. The notification message will prompt the preparation of specific equipment. For the patient with a closed head injury and reduced level of response, prepare and check equipment for intubation; for the patient who has been stabbed in the chest, prepare equipment for a chest drain (and have the emergency thoracotomy set to hand).

Drugs. It takes time to draw up drugs, which will divert the nursing staff from availability for other tasks in the resuscitation. Injured patients who are conscious are invariably in pain: draw up analgesia in advance (for example, morphine 10 mg in 10 mL) and an antiemetic. Where intubation is predictable, draw up the drugs for a rapid sequence induction of anaesthesia (in units that deal with a high turnover of trauma these drugs may be drawn up routinely between trauma cases). Run through intravenous fluids (for example, 1 L crystalloid). Order universal donor blood if critical hypovolaemia is anticipated (see Rule 30).

Space. Arrange the bedspace so there is enough room for easy access of the ambulance trolley. Position three of the team on the far side of the emergency department (ED) trolley who will assist in rapid transfer of the patient. Position the mobile X-ray unit (or gantry unit) next to the trolley and place the chest film plate in the trolley's cassette. Where a child is expected and the age is known, calculate the doses of common drugs in advance (analgesia, glucose, fluid bolus) using the formula weight (kg) = $[2 \times (\text{age in years} + 4)]$.

The exceptions

Preparation is not always possible. Experience will demonstrate to you that organization is improved and anxiety is reduced when there has been adequate time to prepare.

If in doubt, call the Trauma Team

The reason

It is natural to be concerned about your ability to manage a seriously injured patient when your experience is limited. When you stop being concerned about your abilities and become complacent is the time to worry. But you should never be afraid to ask for help.

In many hospitals, the Trauma Team will be activated according to established criteria, based on the history of the incident, the anatomical injury and the observed vital signs [6]. Example activation criteria are as follow.

History
- Fall >5 m
- Pedestrian or cyclist hit by a vehicle
- Other occupant killed
- Ejected from vehicle

Injuries
- >1 long bone fractured (radius and ulna on the same side count as 1)
- >1 anatomical area injured
- Penetrating injury to the torso or head
- >15% burns (>10% in child)
- Traumatic amputation or crush injury

Vital signs
- Respiratory rate >29/minute
- Pulse rate >130 or <50/minute
- Systolic BP <90 mmHg
- Glasgow Coma Scale <13

In the military environment there is often limited information on casualties before arrival at the field hospital: the decision to activate the Trauma Team may be based solely on whether the casualty is categorized 'Priority 1' ('Immediate'/'T1') in the alerting message (see Rule 67).

The exceptions

When the Trauma Team is activated on mechanism of injury alone (the history), there will be a significant proportion of cases where no serious pathology is found [7]. This could be regarded as the price to pay for not missing those with serious occult injury; however, some institutions utilize a two-tier trauma response to significantly limit over-triage [8–10] or initial assessment by an emergency physician where there are no abnormal physiological or anatomical indicators following *blunt* trauma [11]. Activation criteria based on physiology are likely to lead to an over-estimation of a child's severity of injury (see Rule 67).

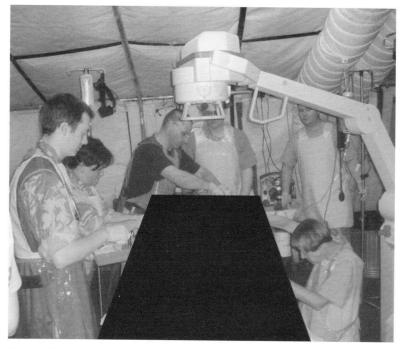

Figure 6.1 Personal protective equipment.

Save yourself before the casualty

The reason
All trauma patients should be considered a high risk for blood transmissible diseases, particularly the HIV and hepatitis viruses.

REMEMBER
Think of your safety to begin,
When infected you're no use to him.

Personal protective equipment for the resuscitation room should include:
- Eye protection (goggles/safety glasses/visor/face-shield)
- Impervious gown or apron
- Latex gloves
- Lead apron

When there is advanced warning, the team should be appropriately dressed before the patient arrives. Equipment is ideally stored by the entrance to the resuscitation area to encourage staff to put on the equipment before approaching the patient.

Personal protective equipment is primarily to protect *you* from the *patient*. However, if you as a healthcare worker have a transmissible disease you have an ethical, and in some cases a legal, responsibility to declare this or remove yourself from the environment where you may come into contact with the injured.

The exceptions
It is common for staff to enter the resuscitation area after the seriously injured patient has arrived and treatment has started. **Always** pause to take suitable precautions to protect yourself from a patient's bodily fluids before you give treatment.

The greatest protection from radiation is distance and for non-essential staff to remove themselves from the resuscitation area when a radiograph is exposed. Essential staff can and should stay with the patient to continue care, provided that they wear protective lead gowns.

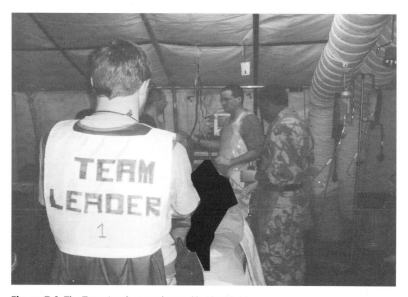

Figure 7.1 The Team Leader must be readily identifiable.

The Team Leader is always right

The reason

For a Trauma Team to run effectively there must be an identifiable leader who will direct the resuscitation, assess the priorities and make critical decisions [12]. Members of the team must respect this authority and be prepared to carry out the leader's instructions.

Strong leadership will instil a sense that the best possible outcome was achieved, even when the patient dies; weak leadership will induce anxiety and frustration in the team members, even when there is a positive outcome.

Team leadership is increasingly the role of the emergency physician. However, it is the competencies that determine a leader rather than their appointment. Effective leadership requires a sound knowledge of trauma resuscitation consolidated through experience; an ability to analyse the array of physical findings and make a judgement on priorities for investigation and treatment; an understanding of the specialist resources available locally and regionally that may be accessed for definitive care; and the ability to communicate both clearly and with authority.

The Team Leader is optimally situated at the foot of the bed and is not responsible for interventional skills (securing an airway; chest drain; intravenous access). Should interventional skills be carried out by the Team Leader then the ability to control the team can be lost.

The Team Leader needs to be readily identifiable. In large hospitals where the team membership changes daily and there is an element of staff unfamiliarity, it is useful for tabards (vests) to be worn that identify roles (Figure 7.1). When it is necessary for leadership to change (for example, on the arrival of a more senior doctor during a difficult resuscitation) then the tabard should be handed over.

The exceptions

A good Team Leader will support and encourage the team, will seek advice from other expert members of the team and will allow their instructions to be questioned. The Team Leader cannot always be right, but after discussion the leader **must** make the final decision.

Approach to the patient

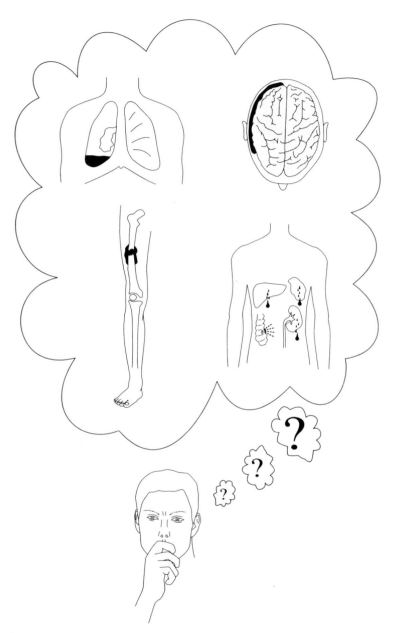

Figure 8.1 Assume the worst and proceed accordingly.

Assume the worst and proceed accordingly

The reason

Every patient who fulfils the criteria to activate the Trauma Team should be treated in the same manner. Do not be tempted to take short-cuts in the primary survey.

The disadvantage of adopting a rigid protocol for all trauma victims is that a proportion will be over-treated, will have undergone invasive procedures (venous cannulation, rectal and vaginal examination, urinary catheterization) and will have been exposed to radiation without any significant injury being discovered. Some may even be discharged home from the resuscitation room. This is the price for not missing those who do have significant but initially occult injury, suggested by the mechanism of injury rather than the anatomical injury or the physiological signs at the scene of injury.

The exceptions

Only substantial clinical experience in trauma management can justify any short-cuts to the assessment and treatment of trauma victims.

Read the wreckage

The reason

Blunt injuries following a motor vehicle crash may be predicted by *reading the wreckage*. Is it a front impact, a side impact or a roll-over? Each has a characteristic pattern of injuries. The injuries that can be anticipated from a front impact are given as an example:

* *Head and face:* if no restraint is worn, the face may 'bulls-eye' the windscreen resulting in facial fractures and internal head injuries. The head may also strike the rear view mirror.

* *Cervical spine:* the neck is subject to flexion and extension forces with consequent ligamentous injury and fractures.

* *Chest:* if no restraint is worn, severe chest injuries may result from impact with the steering wheel (where no airbag deploys). Suspect rib fractures, a central flail, pulmonary injury and cardiac contusion. If restraint is worn, clavicle and sternal injuries are commonly seen.

* *Abdomen:* compression of the abdomen from the steering wheel may result in diaphragmatic rupture (usually the left hemi-diaphragm); bruising across the abdomen from seatbelt tensioning should raise the suspicion of hollow viscus injury (for example, small bowel perforation).

* *Pelvis:* compression of the femur by an intruding dashboard may dislocate the hip posteriorly (look for a hip with a fixed flexion deformity and an abducted, internally rotated thigh)—be suspicious if there is patellar injury.

* *Lower limbs:* intrusion of the engine compartment may cause tibia/fibula injuries. Feet may be trapped by deformed pedals (release may be possible by cutting the boot laces and pulling the foot free).

The rate of deceleration is important. A motorcyclist who has fallen off and is separated from his or her bike by 50 m has exchanged energy less abruptly than one who has collided at the same speed with a wall and is found next to the bike.

A digital (or Polaroid) photograph taken at the scene can provide an appreciation of the mechanism which is often inadequately understood by the receiving hospital staff. Virtually all patients arrive at hospital lying on their back on a long spinal board. This does not convey the likelihood of injury that may be clear to the rescuers dealing with a complex entrapment.

The same principle applies to a casualty with burns who has escaped by jumping out of a window, or a springboard diver who floats to the surface of the pool after striking his or her head (and flexing his or her neck) on the pool bottom.

The exceptions

Injuries may be ameliorated by wearing a seatbelt, by airbags and by side impact protection systems such that the occupant can walk away relatively unscathed even when the vehicle deformation suggests the potential for serious injury. Penetrating injuries cannot be reliably predicted simply by observing the scene, although the pattern of entry and exit wounds can be suggestive (but can also mislead).

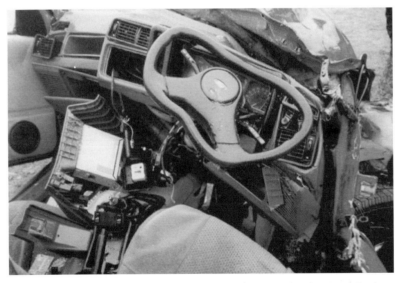

Figure 9.1 Reading the wreckage. What injuries would you suspect in the unrestrained driver of this vehicle?

Do a frisk or take a risk

The reason

Do not assume that a patient who has been shot or stabbed is an innocent victim of an unprovoked crime. There may have been a two-way exchange of violence and the patient may be carrying a weapon.

Hypoxia causes confusion and aggression. Do not give the hypoxic patient the opportunity of confusing you with an aggressor. Do a rapid frisk for weapons and make them safe. If you do not know how to make a firearm safe, place it on the floor out of the way and have it guarded until the police arrive.

It is standard practice within a field hospital to ensure the removal of all weapons and pyrotechnics before the patient enters the hospital complex.

Alleged relatives of local civilians admitted to a field hospital on overseas operations require searching for weapons, unless the role of the hospital is humanitarian in support of a natural disaster.

The exceptions

An armed assailant who has been injured during apprehension by the police will already have been frisked for weapons.

Don't let the obvious distract from the occult

The reason

An immediately obvious injury may distract you from a less obvious but life-threatening injury. This is particularly likely with orthopaedic injuries—for example, a major joint dislocation, angulated long-bone fracture or partial amputation will distract your attention, but will you immediately notice the obstructed airway or tension pneumothorax?

For this reason, it is always wise to follow a systematic approach to assessment and management of an injured patient.

The exceptions

Some obvious injuries are life-threatening: for example, a traumatic limb amputation with arterial haemorrhage. In this situation it is common sense to arrest the haemorrhage rapidly before proceeding through the ABC assessment. Remember that a Trauma Team works horizontally, with all critical systems being assessed and treated simultaneously [13]. It is only when you are on your own that you must work vertically and attend to <C> then A then B then C.

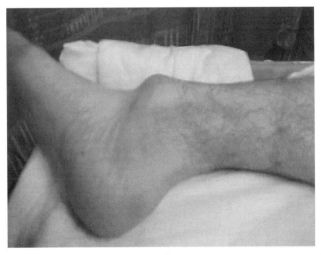

Figure 11.1 Don't let the obvious distract from the occult: there is a dislocation of the ankle which requires urgent reduction—but is there a more pressing priority first?

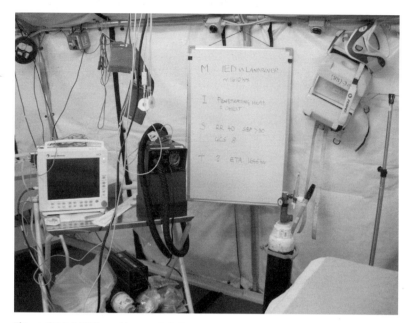

Figure 12.1 MIST board to record alert message.

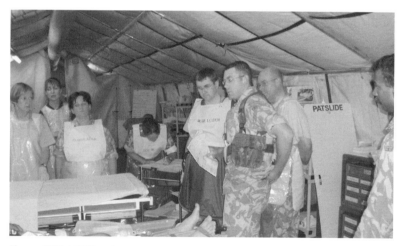

Figure 12.2 MIST handover.

The Trauma Team can only look or listen, not both

The reason

It is a common observation that the Trauma Team fails to absorb the information from the ambulance paramedic during the handover of the patient. This is because the human being is essentially a single channel processor, and the doctor who is concentrating on assessing the patient cannot also concentrate on the spoken information from the paramedic.

One way to address this problem is for the whole trauma team to stand and listen to the patient handover before anyone approaches the patient [14]. The paramedic is given up to 45 seconds to describe:

M Mechanism of injury
I Injuries found and suspected
S Signs (respiratory rate, oxygen saturation, pulse rate, blood pressure)
T Treatment given

This is time well spent: it will reduce unnecessary repetition of the story and will prevent vital information being lost. It is useful to have a board in the resuscitation room on which to write this information, placed where anyone else entering the room can see it.

The exceptions

The Trauma Team will not wait for a handover if basic life support is in progress, or if the airway is obstructed. In this case, the Team Leader should instruct the ambulance crew to wait for an opportunity to pass the pre-hospital information.

Initial assessment and resuscitation

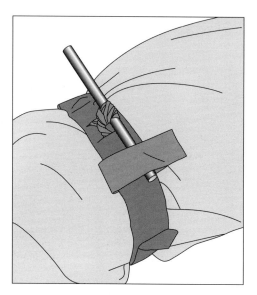

Figure 13.1 A one-handed military tourniquet.

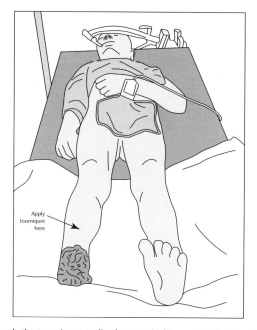

Apply
tourniquet
here

Figure 13.2 Apply the tourniquet as distal as practical to control the bleeding.

Tourniquets save lives

The reason

Tourniquets have become a victim of irrational taboo. In an analysis of US military deaths in Vietnam, there were more than 2500 who died from limb injuries alone; it has been extrapolated that 7% of battlefield deaths could have been prevented by the application of a tourniquet.

More recently, an analysis of 550 Israeli victims of military trauma (1997–2001) revealed that no casualty died from uncontrolled limb bleeding when a tourniquet was used. One or more tourniquets were applied for life-threatening limb bleeding in 91 cases, but 0 of the 125 deaths in this series had a tourniquet applied [15]. Some required multiple tourniquets for injuries to two or even three limbs, and some limbs had more than one tourniquet applied. If the bleeding was not controlled by the first tourniquet, a second was placed proximally. This supports the assertion that *tourniquets save lives*.

The value of an improvised tourniquet has been undermined by evidence that it takes a trained military medic over 4 minutes to apply an improvised device effectively [16]. This should be interpreted in the context of a total blood volume of 5 L and a loss of 1 L/minute through a severed femoral artery [17].

A commercial tourniquet that can be applied rapidly is required to arrest catastrophic haemorrhage from major vessels in the limbs. Tourniquets that can be applied with one hand have become popular in the military (Figure 13.1) to allow the soldier to self-apply a tourniquet before passing out through hypovolaemia and to continue to fight, at least for a short time.

In most situations, a tourniquet should be left *in situ* once it has been applied. Where it has been applied under fire, it is reasonable to attempt a trial without tourniquet once the fire-fight has been won. It is important to record the *time* that the tourniquet was applied (on the pre-hospital record, the triage label or the casualty's forehead).

The exceptions

A tourniquet is applied because limb haemorrhage cannot be controlled by any other means. You are effectively choosing to sacrifice the limb below the level of the tourniquet in order to save the life. Apply the tourniquet as distal as is practical in order to control the haemorrhage (Figure 13.2).

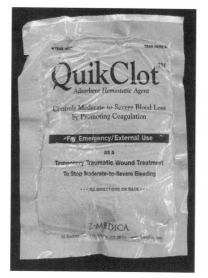
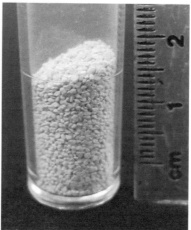

Figure 14.1 *QuikClot™.*

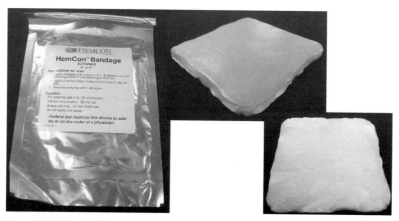

Figure 14.2 *HemCon™.*

If the bleeding is dramatic, use a novel haemostatic

The reason

The high casualty rate sustained by US forces in the aftermath of the Second Gulf War precipitated an aggressive research programme to identify topical haemostatic agents for use in massive external haemorrhage that could not be controlled effectively by direct pressure or the use of a tourniquet (for example, groin or axilla wounds involving major vessels).

Two agents have dominated the military market, although additional agents in development are expected to challenge for the position as the preferred topical haemostatic.

QuikClot™ (zeolite; Figure 14.1) is derived from volcanic rock and is an inert powder. It is designed to be poured into the wound, although the wound bowl should be mopped of excess blood using a dressing in order to limit the significant heat generated on contact with blood. Free powder must be brushed away immediately from the lips of the wound to prevent a cutaneous burn. HemCon™ (chitosan; Figure 14.2) is an active dressing that is capable of sealing high-volume high-pressure arterial injury and works by ionic attraction of red blood cells (independently of whether there are clotting factors present or hypothermia, both of which may be present in the polytraumatized patient). Both agents have been shown to be highly effective in large animal models simulating major vessel injury and in military case series [18]. Pressure is required for 3 minutes over the wound in both cases following application.

The use of novel haemostatics is part of the strategy to reduce avoidable deaths from haemorrhage in conflict situations. External haemorrhage is the most common avoidable cause of death in this environment and is the driver to modify the **ABC** paradigm to **<C>ABC** (where **<C>** is **catastrophic haemorrhage**; see Rule 1).

The exceptions

QuikClot™ in its powder form is unsuitable to place into a wound with pulsatile bleeding (as the agent will be ejected onto the skin surface, potentially resulting in a burn). In a second generation formulation the powder has been placed inside a porous bag to overcome this limitation.

HemCon™ in its original formulation was a stiff 10 × 10 cm bandage, which is unsuitable for narrow entrance wounds. In a second generation formulation it has been developed as a ribbon gauze.

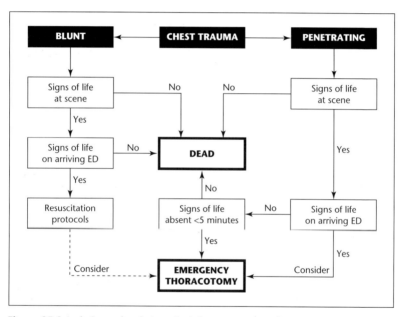

Figure 15.1 Inclusion and exclusion criteria for an emergency thoracotomy following chest trauma. ED, emergency department.

If you decide to crack the chest, survival's almost nil at best

The reason

The outcome following cardiac arrest secondary to trauma is universally poor. Where there are no vital signs at the scene following *blunt trauma*, then survival at hospital approaches 0%. Where a thoracotomy is performed within 5 minutes of losing vital signs following *penetrating trauma*, there is a variable chance of survival, dependent on the protocols used and the expertise of the unit. Survival following emergency thoracotomy for a stab wound is substantially greater than for a gunshot wound [19].

For this reason cardiopulmonary resuscitation (*basic life support*, BLS) is inappropriate following traumatic cardiac arrest in the battlefield setting. Moving a body with BLS in progress in this context places an unnecessary risk on the medical services. It achieves nothing other than changing the geographical site of death and shifting the level of responsibility at which death is pronounced.

The exceptions

The outcome from cardiac arrest secondary to *ischaemic heart disease* is related to early BLS and early defibrillation; these are routinely performed as external techniques.

Emergency thoracotomy may be justifiable when vital signs are lost and there is immediate access to surgical intervention. This may be performed in the emergency department or an adjacent operating theatre (in the field hospital the operating theatre is adjacent to the emergency department). This intervention is also taught to pre-hospital doctors who provide the helicopter emergency medical services (HEMS) in the UK. Appropriate patient selection is essential, with the following used as a guide:

Penetrating trauma	Witnessed cardiac arrest with immediate surgical access
	Unresponsive hypotension (systolic blood pressure <70 mmHg)
Blunt trauma	Unresponsive hypotension (systolic blood pressure <70 mmHg)
	Rapid exsanguination from chest tube (>1500 mL)

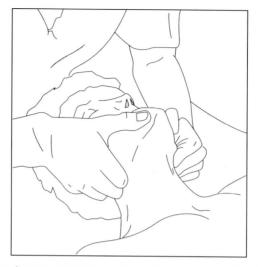

Figure 16.1 Jaw thrust to open the airway (the preferred manoeuvre following blunt trauma).

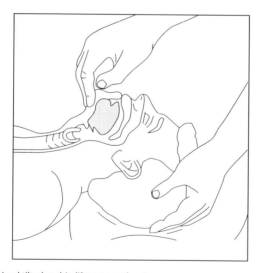

Figure 16.2 Head tilt plus chin lift to open the airway.

The airway is more important than the cervical spine

The reason
The judgement to immobilize the cervical spine is often based on the mechanism of injury rather than the presence of symptoms and signs indicating spinal injury [20]. The cervical spine is therefore usually immobilized because of **potential** injury, not absolute injury. However, airway obstruction is an **absolute** problem: if untreated the patient will certainly die.

In general, the airway is opened and secured while stabilizing the cervical spine—but when there is impending death from airway obstruction, protection of the cervical spine is not the priority [21]. Actions may include tilting of the head to obtain a clear airway.

Every effort should be made to *maximize success of the first attempt at intubation*. This will include removal of straps and head-blocks for those secured on a long spinal board and loosening or removal of the semi-rigid cervical collar: this sequence is carried out while manual in-line stabilization is maintained. Additionally, all equipment and drugs are prepared (and some prefer to 'preload' the endotracheal tube with a gum elastic bougie during *every* rapid sequence induction of anaesthesia), the patient is pre-oxygenated and there is assistance to maintain cricoid pressure during the procedure [22].

The exceptions
Even in the presence of clinical signs of spinal injury, the airway must take priority. In any case, the patient who most benefits from immobilization is the one **without** neurological symptoms. If there are symptoms, the damage has been done already and is unlikely to be made worse by the pre-hospital handling or handling in the resuscitation room.

When NEXUS guidelines clear the spine, the spinal board's a waste of time

The reason

NEXUS Guidelines from the USA (National Emergency X-radiograph Utilization Study, with guidelines validated on >30 000 patients) [23] are an established framework for clinical clearance of the cervical spine following blunt trauma (99% sensitivity for detecting a fracture). The cervical spine can be cleared if:

- The patient is Glasgow Coma Scale (GCS) 15 (normal level of alertness) *and*
- There is no posterior mid-line tenderness *and*
- There is no distracting injury (other painful injury) *and*
- There is no focal neurological deficit *and*
- There is no intoxication (alcohol or drugs, including iatrogenic)

Cervical spine X-rays should be performed on all other patients (Figure 17.1). Three-view plain X-ray imaging (lateral, AP, peg) is recommended for conscious patients (sensitivity of ~94% for showing fracture in symptomatic patients). A swimmer's view is performed if C7–T1 junction is not seen on the lateral view. If these images are normal, the casualty can be clinically examined and cervical spine precautions removed if he or she is non-tender and demonstrates a full range of active neck movements. If there is mid-line tenderness, flexion and extension films are used to assess for ligamentous injury.

The **level of motor deficit** is taken as the lowest muscle with power of 3/5 (American Spinal Injury Association Scale, where grade 3 power is a full range of movement against gravity). The **level of sensory deficit** is taken as the lowest dermatome bilaterally to have normal sensation.

When CT is available, it is appropriate to image the lower cervical spine if not seen on plain X-ray. When CT of the brain is undertaken following blunt trauma, it is recommended to extend the imaging to include C1–3.

CT with reconstructed images of the cervical spine is increasingly used in trauma centres as a primary imaging tool for the head-injured patient sent to CT for brain imaging (i.e. US practice is to defer plain cervical spine radiographs in favour of CT imaging for head-injured patients).

Spinal cord injury without radiological abnormality (SCIWORA) is a rare phenomenon (0.08% of cervical spine injuries) that occurs in both adults and children. The most common injuries (magnetic resonance imaging, MRI, confirmation) are central disc herniation, spinal stenosis and cord oedema or contusion.

Penetrating spinal injuries from military weaponry may be destructive and are generally contaminated. Even if the round or fragment does not directly hit the spinal cord, bony secondary fragments can cause injury and the effects of cavitation or blast result in microscopically detectable injury centimetres distant to the track of the round. There is no evidence that spinal immobilization limits further injury following penetrating trauma.

The exceptions

Full spinal immobilization following blunt trauma may still be inappropriate when cervical spine injury cannot be ruled out if:

1 The patient has a facial injury that results in airway obstruction when they lie flat: the conscious patient is best managed initially in the sitting position.

2 The patient is combative (from head injury and/or hypoxia) and struggles when actively restrained by the head-blocks and/or cervical collar.

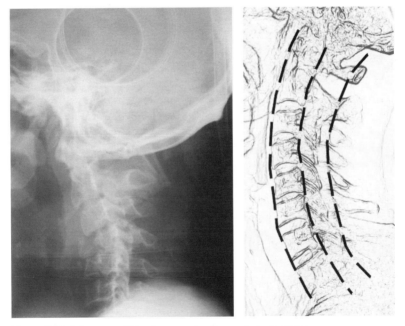

Figure 17.1 Follow your ABCs when assessing the cervical spine X-ray.

A, adequacy and alignment. Can you see all seven vertebrae and C7–T1 junction? Is there normal alignment?

B, Bones. Trace around the contour of each vertebral body and spinous process.

C, Cartilages. Look at the spaces between the facet joints and the spaces between the vertebrae.

S, soft tissues. Check the spaces between the peg and anterior arch of C1; look for an increased soft tissue space anterior to the vertebral bodies (indicating occult bleeding).

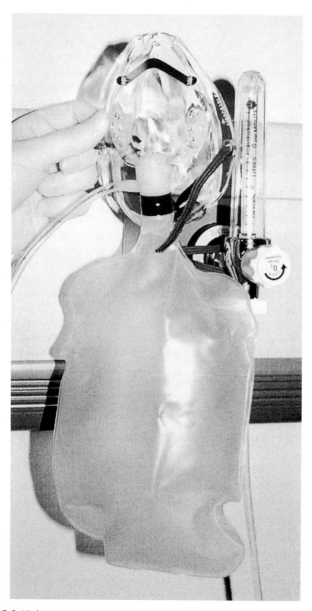

Figure 18.1 High-concentration oxygen can be delivered through a tight-fitting face mask with attached reservoir.

All trauma patients are dying for oxygen

The reason

All patients with significant trauma will have a degree of hypoxia as a result of airway compromise, chest injury, hypoventilation from head injury, or hypovolaemia. To improve oxygen delivery to hypoxic tissues, all victims of trauma should be given high-concentration oxygen [24]. When spontaneously breathing, the best delivery system is a tight-fitting Hudson face-mask with an attached reservoir bag and oxygen at 10–15 L/min, adjusted to the minimum flow required to keep the reservoir bag inflated (Figure 18.1). This provides an inspired oxygen concentration in excess of 85% (FiO_2 >0.85).

If ventilation is being assisted, 100% oxygen can be delivered through a bag-valve device (attached to a mask or endotracheal tube), when a reservoir bag is incorporated into the system and the oxygen flow is adjusted between 10 and 15 L/min to keep the reservoir inflated.

However, remember that *oxygen is free—so don't make your patients work for it!* This refers to the increased work of breathing to draw oxygen through a bag-valve-mask apparatus than a Hudson mask: reserve the bag-valve-mask for assisted ventilation or pre-oxygenation immediately prior to intubation.

The exceptions

It is essential to give all victims of significant trauma supplemental high-concentration oxygen, even those patients with chronic lung disease [25]. They are all hypoxic, and hypoxia is compounded if there is chronic lung disease. If respiration is suppressed, ventilation can be assisted. **CO_2 kills slowly, but no O_2 kills quickly**.

Oxygen may not be available in the military environment or it may be in limited supply, requiring its use to be prioritized and/or lower flow rates used. The flow rate in trauma is cited as 15 L/min, but this can be reduced to a rate that is adequate to keep the reservoir bag partially inflated on inspiration and still ensure a high O_2 concentration.

REMEMBER
A is for airway with cervical spine **where appropriate**
B is for breathing with oxygen **where available**

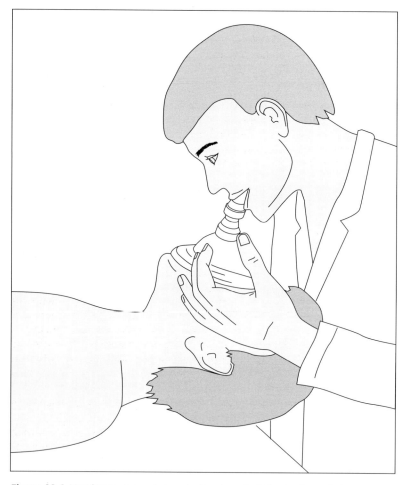

Figure 19.1 Ventilation via a pocket mask: do not overlook the simple ventilation techniques.

It is not lack of intubation that kills, it is lack of oxygenation

The reason

Assisted ventilation may be required because of *hypoventilation* (as a result of the injury or respiratory depressant drugs, such as opiates used for analgesia), because of *ineffective ventilation* (for example, with a flail chest and underlying contusion) or in *traumatic cardiac arrest*.

A bag-valve-mask apparatus is often sufficient in the pre-hospital or early hospital resuscitation phases to provide oxygenation. Intubation can usually only be attempted in the pre-hospital setting when the patient is completely unresponsive, as generally there is no access to intravenous anaesthetic and paralysing agents. Should intubation be attempted outside hospital, it is important that the patient is pre-oxygenated before each attempt and that professional pride does not prevent the paramedic reverting to a simpler technique. Equally, the bag-valve-mask technique can be difficult with one operator (two operators are ideal, with one to hold the mask with both hands and one to ventilate) and the operator should not be afraid to discard the bag-valve-mask in favour of a *Laerdal Pocket Mask™*. **It is better to deliver 17% expired air oxygen to the lungs than to deliver 100% oxygen to the back of the mouth**.

The *Laryngeal Mask Airway* (LMA) and the *Combi-tube™* are advanced airway adjuncts that can be positioned blind (without the need for a laryngoscope) by medical, paramedical or nursing staff after relatively little training. The devices allow ventilation via a bag-valve device, but in general do not provide the same degree of airway protection as a cuffed endotracheal tube. The LMA has found particular favour in UK clinical use and a high proportion of anaesthetics for surgery are administered with an LMA: this gives considerable opportunity for training and skills maintenance. While limited studies favoured the *Combi-tube™* for use by paramedics, it has not become an established standard.

The exceptions

A patient with a head injury who is comatose (Glasgow Coma Scale <9) on arrival at hospital requires early endotracheal intubation to protect the airway, to provide a reliable route of supplying high-concentration oxygen to limit secondary brain damage and to control the partial pressure of carbon dioxide (CO_2). In this case, it is reasonable to aim for intubation within 10 minutes of arrival in the resuscitation room. It is vital to pre-oxygenate the patient before each intubation attempt.

Oesophageal intubation is predictable occasionally, even in the most experienced hands. It may be detected by inadequate chest movement or air entry on positive pressure ventilation, or by end-tidal CO_2 monitoring (digital reading or colorimetric disposable device). **It is not negligent to intubate the oesophagus—it is only negligent to fail to recognize it has occurred**.

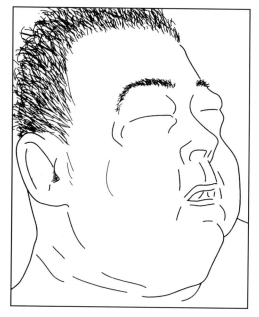

Figure 20.1 Anticipate obstruction of the airway with facial oedema following burns. Do not delay with a burned airway.

Do not delay with a burned airway

The reason

Laryngeal oedema secondary to inhalational burns develops very rapidly, often within minutes, and can present the anaesthetist with one of the most difficult intubations they are likely to face. The following signs indicate the presence of upper airway burns and the need to consider early elective intubation:

- Respiratory distress
- Burns around the mouth
- Oedema of the face or lips
- Oropharyngeal carbon or carbonaceous sputum
- Singed nasal hairs
- Inflammation, oedema or blistering of the oropharynx or tongue
- Hoarse voice

In the early period following a burn that involves the upper airway the patient may walk and talk at the scene and have relatively normal physiology. Although the triage category for treatment at the scene would be low in these circumstances (see Rule 67), the highest priority must be given for evacuation of patients with suspected upper airway burns from the scene; these patients are potentially salvageable. Delay may be very costly.

When there are inhalational burns, always consider concomitant carbon monoxide (CO) poisoning. The principal treatment for CO poisoning is high-concentration oxygen. Hyperbaric oxygen should be considered in the following circumstances:

- Loss of consciousness at scene
- Carboxyhaemoglobin levels >30% (this threshold may vary between hyperbaric units and should be checked locally)
- Pregnancy
- Presence of focal neurological signs

The exceptions

Flash burns will often cause superficial burns and singeing of the eyebrows and hair, but may not involve the upper airway. Look for the suggestive signs of additional upper airway burn listed above.

While hyperbaric oxygen will greatly reduce the half-life of carboxyhaemoglobin (to approximately 20 minutes), the benefit of this treatment must be balanced against the need for other life-saving treatment, such as surgery for injuries incurred during an escape from the fire. The hyperbaric unit may be no more than a coffin-sized chamber and, if complications arise during treatment, intervention to treat them can be difficult. If the patient requires an endotracheal tube the cuff should be filled with water, otherwise it will deflate and the tube may become dislodged.

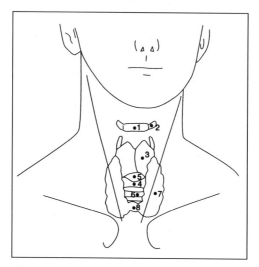

Figure 21.1 Anatomy of the larynx. 1 Body of the hyoid cartilage. 2 Greater horn of hyoid cartilage. 3 Thyroid cartilage. 4 Cricoid cartilage. 5 Cricothyroid membrane. 6 Tracheal ring. 7 Lobe of thyroid. 8 Thyroid isthmus.

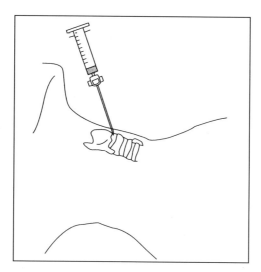

Figure 21.2 Needle cricothyrotomy technique.

Think of cricothyrotomy when all else fails

The reason

Cricothyrotomy is a means of bypassing an obstructed upper airway when all other means of obtaining an airway have failed, including manual manoeuvres (chin lift or jaw thrust), simple airway adjuncts (oropharyngeal and nasopharyngeal airway) and endotracheal intubation [26].

Cricothyrotomy may occasionally be necessary in the trauma resuscitation room with upper airway obstruction secondary to a foreign body or oedema (from burns, facial fractures or, rarely, anaphylaxis from drugs administered).

A *needle cricothyrotomy* involves inserting a large-bore cannula through the cricothyroid membrane. Then, with a Y-connector (or tubing with a side hole), jet-insufflating oxygen from a cylinder or wall source at 15 L/minute [27]. A *surgical cricothyrotomy* requires an incision in the cricothyroid membrane, through which a cuffed tracheostomy-type tube can be inserted. The minimal definitive airway for an adult is 6 mm internal diameter.

> The threshold for undertaking a surgical airway will be lower in the military environment and will be influenced by the non-availability far forward of drugs or the skills to secure the airway under anaesthesia and the prolonged evacuation times during which intervention can be extremely difficult (for example, in a helicopter that is flying tactically).
>
> The open technique (an incision in the cricothyroid membrane) is preferred in this environment to a closed Seldinger needle procedure because of reliability and the degree of dexterity demanded. Comprehensive kits are commercially available to assist the open procedure in a crisis.

A principal complication of cricothyrotomy is to insert the needle or the tube anterior to the membrane, subcutaneously. When assisted ventilation is started, the neck will distend with massive surgical emphysema and landmarks will be lost.

The exceptions

In children under 12 years, a surgical cricothyrotomy is not recommended. This is because the tracheal cartilage rings are immature and the support for the upper trachea is provided by the cricoid cartilage. When the cricothyroid membrane is incised this support can be lost.

A tracheostomy is not a technique for the emergency room. It requires a skilled surgeon, is more time consuming and has a considerable risk of significant haemorrhage.

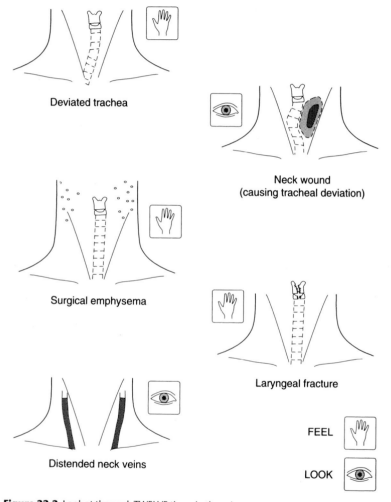

Deviated trachea

Neck wound
(causing tracheal deviation)

Surgical emphysema

Laryngeal fracture

Distended neck veins

FEEL

LOOK

Figure 22.2 Look at the neck TWELVE times in the primary survey.

Look at the neck TWELVE times in the primary survey

The reason

The neck carries the airway and the circulation to the brain. For this reason it is important to examine the neck in the primary survey. It is natural to do this after inspecting the upper airway and before examining the chest. The considerations are as follows:

T	Trachea	If this is deviated, suspect a tension pneumothorax.
W	Wounds	Are there wounds in the neck threatening the airway or circulation? Do not probe these wounds in the emergency department.
E	Emphysema	Surgical emphysema in the neck may suggest a disrupted airway or a pneumothorax.
L	Larynx	Is the larynx intact? If not, the airway is in immediate danger.
V	Veins	Distended neck veins suggest a tension pneumothorax or cardiac tamponade.
E	Every time	*Don't forget* to look at the neck before you put on the semi-rigid cervical collar. With the collar in place you may miss these important signs.

The exceptions

A semi-rigid cervical collar is usually in place when a blunt trauma victim arrives at hospital, often with additional cervical spine support (head-blocks and securing straps). Many semi-rigid collars still allow limited examination of the neck through a cut-away section anteriorly. Unless there is a suspicion of a life-threatening injury in the neck, the collar should not be removed routinely in the primary survey, but will be removed as part of the secondary survey while maintaining manual immobilization of the cervical spine.

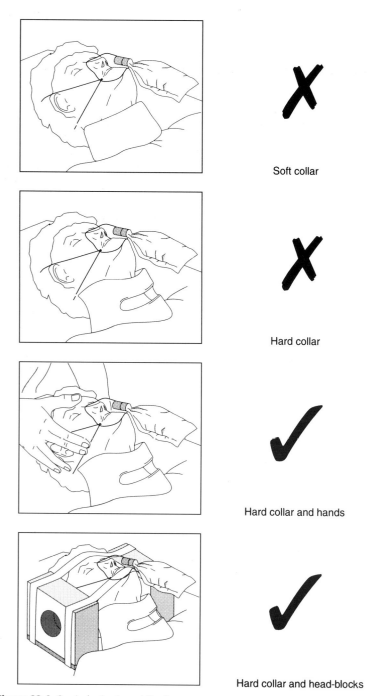

Soft collar

Hard collar

Hard collar and hands

Hard collar and head-blocks

Figure 23.1 Cervical spine immobilization.

A hard collar does not protect the cervical spine

The reason

A soft collar does not protect the cervical spine—it will simply keep the neck warm.

A hard collar (also referred to as a *semi-rigid collar*) is just a flag that says, 'Protect this neck, it may be injured', and on its own it is also inadequate protection for the cervical spine. A hard collar must be paired with manual in-line stabilization or rigid head immobilization (in head-blocks; or improvised with a rolled blanket in a horseshoe around the head + tape, or the traditional 'sandbags + tape').

Following blunt multisystem trauma, the cervical spine should be assumed to be injured until this has been excluded radiologically and clinically. A high index of suspicion is particularly important with significant other injury above the clavicle.

At the cervical level, the spinal cord occupies approximately 50% of the spinal canal, the rest of the space being filled with connective tissue and fat. It is therefore possible to cause damage to the cervical spine and narrowing of the canal without causing neurological impairment. Careless handling of the patient during extrication and resuscitation could cause further narrowing and precipitate quadraplegia. Remember that it is the patient **without** neurological symptoms who will benefit most from rigid spinal immobilization in the resuscitation.

The exceptions

If the patient is very agitated (and this is seen in distressed children or in patients with associated head injury) it can be detrimental to rigidly immobilize the head, as the body continues to move. In these cases a collar alone has to suffice, but consider the early use of sedation (as long as there is the capacity to manage the airway should it be compromised) [28].

Penetrating trauma to the neck, such as from a gunshot wound, will produce neurological symptoms immediately following injury. If there are no symptoms, there is no injury.

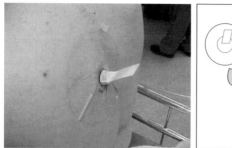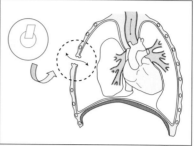

Figure 24.1 Asherman chest seal applied to an open pneumothorax.

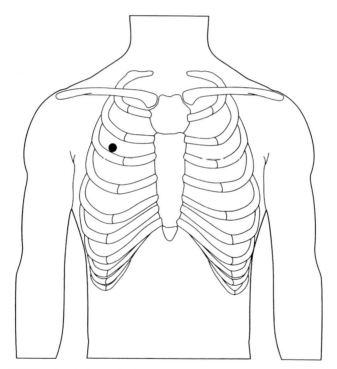

Figure 24.2 Landmarks for needle decompression. Surface markings for needle thoracocentesis. To find the second intercostal space, place your finger at the top of the sternum and move down until you feel a ridge (sternal angle). Now move laterally on to the second rib as far as the mid-clavicular line. Go below the second rib into the second intercostal space. • Second intercostal space, mid-clavicular line.

All Trauma surgeons Occasionally Miss Cervical Fractures

The reason

There are six life-threatening chest conditions that must be considered following trauma. Each of these should be actively sought during the primary survey, and treated immediately when found. The conditions can be remembered as: 'All Trauma surgeons Occasionally Miss Cervical Fractures'.

All	Airway obstruction
Trauma surgeons	Tension pneumothorax
Occasionally	Open pneumothorax
Miss	Massive haemothorax
Cervical	Cardiac tamponade
Fractures	Flail chest

> This rule holds for conventional trauma. In the military context, blast lung must be considered as a life-threatening chest condition. Onset may be immediate, in which case it is often fatal at the scene, or delayed for a period up to many hours.
>
> BLATANTLY All Trauma surgeons Occasionally Miss Cervical Fractures

Only approximately 10% of patients with blunt or penetrating chest injury require thoracotomy, so approximately 90% of chest injuries can be treated by a variable combination of supportive care including chest decompression and drainage, pain control, respiratory support and observation [29].

The exceptions

A clear mechanism of penetrating injury (such as a stab or gunshot wound) will not produce a flail chest.

Inserting a chest drain will treat tension pneumothorax, open pneumothorax and massive haemothorax. However, the immediate treatment for each of these conditions is as follows:

Tension pneumothorax	Needle decompression
Open pneumothorax	Apply chest seal with flutter valve
Massive haemothorax	Start fluids before chest drain

The main treatment for a flail chest is to treat the underlying contusion, which may require ventilatory support. A chest drain would be inserted for an accompanying pneumothorax, and may be appropriate prophylactically with multiple rib fractures before positive pressure ventilation (a small unseen pneumothorax would otherwise tension).

When patients with facial injuries look up at heaven they will soon be there

The reason

Airway obstruction is the principal cause of death with facial injuries [30].

With mid-face fractures (Le Fort fractures) the face may slide posteriorly along the incline of the base of the skull when the patient is supine. A conscious patient with an unstable mid-face will often adopt the most comfortable position for breathing, which is likely to be sitting up and leaning forward. In this position the airway is patent, but will become obstructed if the ambulance officer or emergency physician insists on the patient lying flat.

When the patient is sitting it is important to consider how you will maintain cervical spine integrity—but maintaining the airway is more important than insisting on rigid cervical spinal immobilization in the supine position (see Rule 16).

Airway obstruction with facial injuries may also be a result of heavy bleeding, or from the swelling associated with a fractured jaw.

The exceptions

A patient who is unconscious will be managed in the supine position. The airway can be maintained in the first-aid situation by rolling the patient into the recovery position, but at the risk of inadequately controlling the cervical spine. If the patient is managed in the supine position, the airway may be simply maintained by a combination of suction (to clear aspirated blood), traction on the upper incisors (to pull a shattered mid-face forward) or traction through a transverse tongue suture (when a severely disrupted jaw allows the tongue to fall back into the pharynx).

With a supine patient the cervical spine should be fully immobilized. There is a significant risk of concomitant cervical spine damage with any high-impact blunt injury above the clavicle.

Blood on the floor is lost forever more

The reason

The treatment of bleeding is to stop the bleeding. Why attempt to replace something that you can prevent being lost? Bleeding wounds should therefore be dressed before or at the same time as intravenous access is obtained.

To make a rapid assessment for hidden but significant blood loss on the back of the supine patient, run gloved hands behind the chest and abdomen, and behind the legs. You will need to examine the back of the scalp in the secondary survey as blood loss from scalp wounds can be severe. Remember to look at the sheets and the stretcher: significant blood loss may not have reached the floor.

> The back is conventionally examined in the secondary survey. In penetrating trauma it is essential that the back is examined **early** to exclude a hidden site of significant haemorrhage or an open pneumothorax.

The exceptions

Blood may not be lost forever when the facilities for autotransfusion ('cell saving') exist. This technique was first attempted for trauma in 1886 (in 1818 for postpartum haemorrhage) when Duncan reinfused the blood of a patient whose legs were crushed in a railway incident.

Blood may be outside the circulation for 1–4 hours and still be reinfused (through a micropore filter to remove any debris). A maximum of 3 L autotransfused blood is recommended, and as an adjunct to cross-matched blood. It is particularly valuable in massive haemothorax [31]. The technique is less attractive for intra-abdominal bleeding because of the risk of bacterial contamination, although it can be considered, when available, for isolated solid organ haemorrhage.

Overall, the advantages of autotransfusion are that the blood is immediately available and pre-warmed, there are no transfusion reactions, and the risk of blood-borne infection is eliminated. Also the blood will contain active platelets, normal levels of clotting factors and red blood cells with normal 2,3 DPG levels [32]. The disadvantages are air embolism (very rare in the latest systems), disseminated intravascular coagulopathy and thrombocytopenia.

The technique is not widely used in resuscitation rooms in the UK, perhaps through a combination of cost, absence of technical back-up staff and a lack of familiarity.

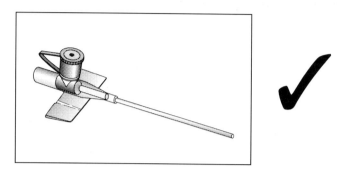

Figure 27.1 Peripheral cannula (14 gauge).

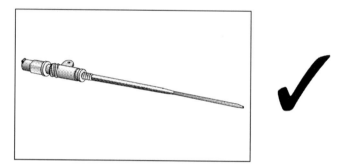

Figure 27.2 Rapid infusion device (7.5 French).

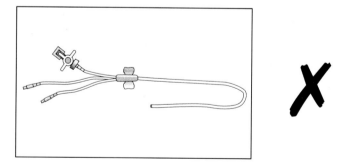

Figure 27.3 Central venous catheter (triple lumen).

Short and thick does the trick

The reason
Do not be fooled into thinking that the patient needs a central line for adequate fluid resuscitation. Flow through a tube is inversely proportional to its length and directly proportional to its radius (to the power of 4). Central lines are often long and thin, whereas peripheral lines are short and thick.

In general, therefore, the patient is best served by fluid resuscitation through a large peripheral cannula. A 16-gauge cannula is not a large peripheral cannula; it is the lower limit of the large range and the minimum size for adequate fluid resuscitation.

The rapid infusion device is a good example of this principle. A short wide-bore cannula (6.5–8.0 French gauge) can be inserted: (a) by percutaneous Seldinger technique (for example, into the femoral vein); (b) by 'rewiring' an existing smaller peripheral cannula (for example, an 18-gauge cannula in the forearm); or (c) directly through an incision in the vein wall during a cut-down (for example, the long saphenous vein).

Remember, flow is not only dependent on the length and radius of the cannula, but also on the viscosity, temperature and pressure of the fluid:

$$\text{Flow} = \frac{P\pi r^4}{8\eta L}$$

where
P = pressure difference
r = radius of the cannula
η = viscosity of the fluid
L = length of the cannula

The exceptions
A Swan–Ganz catheter sheath is placed centrally, usually in the internal jugular vein, but it does have a wide diameter and can be very effective for fluid resuscitation. It should only be inserted by an experienced person, generally an anaesthetist or intensive care specialist.

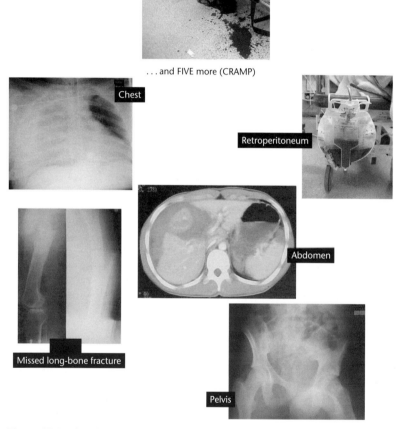

Blood on the floor. . . .

. . . and FIVE more (CRAMP)

Chest

Retroperitoneum

Abdomen

Missed long-bone fracture

Pelvis

Figure 28.1 When there are unexplained signs of bleeding think of blood on the floor and 5 more (CRAMP).

Hidden blood loss will CRAMP your resuscitation

The reason

Signs of blood loss without obvious external haemorrhage include pallor and sweating, tachycardia, tachypnoea, narrow pulse pressure or hypotension, and reduced urinary output. Continuing blood loss is suggested by a failure to respond to intravenous fluid challenges or a non-sustained response.

The following sites of hidden blood loss should be excluded:

C	Chest	Do a chest radiograph
R	Retroperitoneum	Test the urine
A	Abdomen	Do a FAST ultrasound or CT
M	Missed long-bone fracture	Examine the limbs
P	Pelvis	Do a pelvic radiograph

To discover a haemothorax that is not clinically obvious, a chest radiograph is obtained during the primary survey (if the chest X-ray plate is pre-loaded and the Trauma Team is wearing lead gowns the Team Leader states '5...4...3...2...1...chest X-ray!' and it is performed during the primary survey; see Rule 4).

To determine if there is retroperitoneal bleeding, the urine is examined for macroscopic or microscopic blood. Macroscopic blood requires further investigation (structural changes are best seen on a CT scan, whereas function is best assessed with an intravenous urogram).

Intra-abdominal bleeding is suggested by tenderness, distension, guarding and rigidity. When intra-abdominal injury is suspected but the signs are equivocal, investigate with FAST ultrasound or CT (see Rule 53).

A long-bone fracture may be missed when the patient is unresponsive or when a spinal cord injury has produced a loss of sensation. These fractures will be detected by careful clinical examination. Equally, a pelvic fracture may be missed in these circumstances, and a pelvic radiograph should also be obtained during the primary survey.

The exceptions

It is also important to consider that external blood loss at the scene may have been underestimated, and that an inadequate response to fluid replacement may simply mean inadequate fluid replacement when there is no continuing blood loss. A severe scalp wound would be a good example (see Rule 38).

Surgery does not follow resuscitation, it is part of resuscitation

The reason

A running tap may keep an unplugged bath filled, but a patient with an exsanguinating injury requires surgery, not just an endless supply of intravenous fluids. The aim of intravenous fluids in this circumstance is to sustain the patient until life-saving surgery can be performed.

The trauma patient who is 'too ill for surgery' will surely die without surgery. It is not appropriate to wait for surgery until a target pulse or blood pressure is reached with intravenous fluids; in some cases this will never be achieved. However, all measures should be taken to try to ensure the patient is adequately volume resuscitated before emergency surgery.

The resuscitation mantra of the 1980s and 1990s has been 2 L warm crystalloid given rapidly through large-bore peripheral lines. In penetrating trauma of the torso, outcome has been found to be compromised when aggressive fluid resuscitation is given before surgery. This has led to the concept of hypotensive resuscitation [33], and a recommendation that crystalloid is given in the pre-hospital and emergency department settings in 250 mL aliquots to maintain a radial pulse (estimated at maintaining the systolic blood pressure >90 mmHg) [34–36]. However, this policy is extrapolated from outcomes within an advanced urban trauma system in the USA [37] and emerging evidence suggests that sustained hypotensive resuscitation (>2 hours) leads to irreversible acidosis. Fluid resuscitation is therefore a balance of risks [38]. Hypotensive resuscitation coupled with rapid evacuation is the optimum target [39,40]. The search for the optimum resuscitation fluid for use in combat casualty care continues [41].

Patients with closed head injury tolerate hypotension badly, which results in a drop in cerebral perfusion pressure and may exacerbate secondary brain injury. Where head injury is the primary or sole injury it is essential that a normal blood pressure is maintained.

The exceptions

A patient who is moved from the emergency department without their airway being secured, without adequate intravenous access and without a supply of intravenous fluids is very vulnerable on the journey to the operating theatre. Although emergency surgery is part of resuscitation, it does not replace the need to start other resuscitative measures in the emergency department.

The stabbed stay stabbed until they reach theatre

The reason

An impaling object may tamponade a blood vessel it has injured. If the object is removed outside the operating theatre, the resultant haemorrhage may be uncontrollable.

A knife is a sharp instrument and can cause as much damage on the way out from cutting as on the way in. Therefore, explore the wound under anaesthetic and control any major blood vessel (slings and/or clamps) before removing the impaling object.

The exceptions

Small impaling objects in anatomically non-vital tissues may be removed with caution in the emergency department.

O Negative is good, but you can have too much of a good thing

The reason

O Rhesus Negative blood is regarded as the universal donor group. Hospitals will keep a small supply of this blood group for emergency administration of untyped blood. This should be reserved for immediately life-threatening haemorrhage (estimated >40% blood volume lost, or >2 L blood lost). Type-specific blood (an intermediate step to a full cross-match) can be released after 5–10 minutes, but a blood sample has to be drawn and transported to the laboratory and a porter on standby for the transfusion blood to be brought back. Experience reveals this will take a minimum of 20 minutes.

Do not give more than 4 units of O Rhesus Negative blood without knowing the patient's blood group.

If more than 4 units of O Rhesus Negative blood is given, then there will be an admixture of blood cells of different groups. This would interfere with any subsequent cross-match. The sample for cross-match would, however, usually be taken on insertion of the intravenous cannula and before any blood is given.

If more than 4 units of O Rhesus Negative blood are given to a non-O patient who then receives a transfusion of their own blood type, there is likely to be a major haemolytic transfusion reaction [42]. The risk of this occurring has been reduced with the transfusion of packed red blood cells rather than whole blood.

The exceptions

If the patient's blood group is O Rhesus Negative, then you should continue to administer this blood group.

O Rhesus Negative blood is a rare commodity. In these circumstances, and when there is critical hypovolaemia, O Rhesus Positive blood may be given, but not to women of child-bearing potential whose Rhesus status is unknown (may result in Rhesus sensitization to subsequent pregnancies). In other words, **think positive about men, but negative about women** [43].

In the event of shortage of minority groups, alternative red cell groups can be used after discussion with the transfusion service.

Patient group	Preferred alternative group
AB RhD Positive	A RhD Positive
AB RhD Negative	AB or A RhD Positive to male/elderly female
	A RhD Negative to young female
A RhD Negative	A RhD Positive to male/elderly female
	O RhD Negative to young female
B RhD Negative	B RhD Positive to male/elderly female
	O RhD Negative to young female

Blood is a very valuable and finite resource in the military operational setting. Efforts to limit blood consumption are important and may include therapeutic intervention (for example, recombinant Factor VIIa). The use of incompletely screened donors for whole blood donation in a time of crisis is now generally regarded as falling unacceptably below best practice standards, but may be authorized in exceptional circumstances.

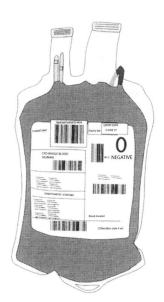

Figure 31.1 O Rhesus Negative is good.

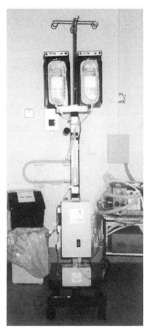

Figure 31.2 All blood should be warm.

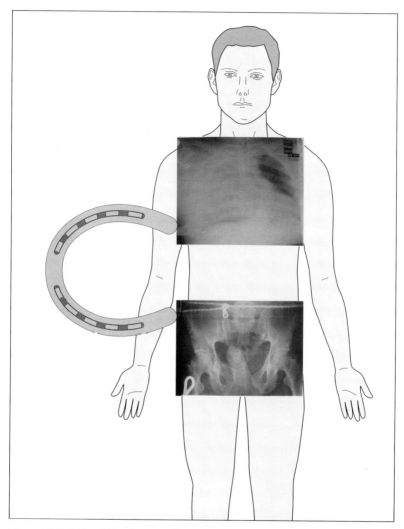

Figure 32.1 A blunt injury above and below the abdomen implies an injury in the abdomen.

An injury above and below the abdomen implies an injury *in* the abdomen . . . unless you have been hit by a giant flying horseshoe!

The reason

The abdomen has little bony protection and its contents are vulnerable. For victims of blunt trauma, especially a motor vehicle accident where there has been diffuse blunt impact (imagine a pedestrian hit by a bus), there should be a high index of suspicion for occult abdominal injury if there are obvious injuries above and below the abdomen.

The exceptions

Penetrating trauma above and below the abdomen does not necessarily indicate injury to the abdomen, although a gunshot wound with an entry in the thigh and exit in the chest must have traversed the abdomen, and a stab wound of the chest can involve the abdomen if the blade was long enough and directed caudally (see Rule 33).

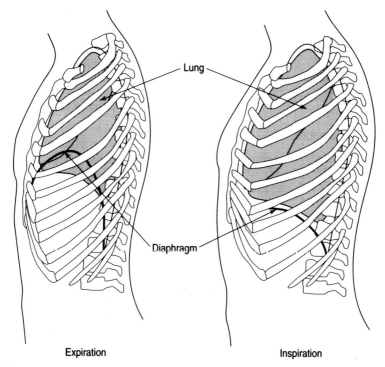

Lung

Diaphragm

Expiration

Inspiration

Figure 33.1 Excursion of the diaphragm during inspiration and expiration. On expiration the diaphragm may rise to the level of the fourth intercostal space anteriorly.

A penetrating wound below the nipple involves the abdomen

The reason

On expiration, the diaphragm will rise anteriorly to approximately the level of the nipple in men. A penetrating wound at or below this level should be presumed to involve the chest and abdominal cavities.

To get into the abdomen from the chest, a penetrating object must pass through the diaphragm. Even in the absence of intra-abdominal visceral injury there may be immediate or delayed rupture of the diaphragm. To exclude diaphragmatic involvement, a laparoscopy or thoracoscopy would be the investigation of choice. Less satisfactorily, or when free intra-peritoneal blood from abdominal visceral involvement is sought, a FAST ultrasound scan (or diagnostic peritoneal lavage, DPL) can be performed in an adult (see Rules 52 & 53). If there is no free blood the patient can be observed and re-examined (with repeat FAST if necessary) at intervals; if there is free blood then surgery is generally required.

Free blood in the abdomen of a child (and in some cases an adult) is not necessarily an indication for surgery, as some visceral injuries can be treated conservatively. A CT scan will define the injury and may allow a conservative approach.

The exceptions

If the patient was stabbed or shot during inspiration, then the injuries may be confined to the chest.

The nipple is not a reliable surface marker in women.

The false negative rate for diagnostic peritoneal lavage with an isolated rupture of the diaphragm is 12–40% for penetrating trauma and 14–36% for blunt trauma. The threshold for operative intervention is therefore reduced to when the red blood cell count is greater than 5×10^6/L in the peritoneal lavage fluid [44].

A conservative approach is only appropriate where there is close observation on an intensive care unit and the opportunity to proceed immediately to surgery if there is deterioration. As a rule, a conservative approach will not be adopted for penetrating trauma of the abdomen in a military setting.

Examination of the abdomen is as reliable as flipping a coin

The reason

The absence of clinical symptoms and signs of peritonism does not reliably exclude free intra-abdominal blood following trauma. In fact, symptoms and signs may be absent in up to 35% of patients [45]. Furthermore, signs may be masked in a patient who is unconscious, intoxicated or who has a high spinal cord injury with loss of abdominal sensation.

In those without symptoms and signs, a high index of suspicion must be maintained, together with close observation of the pulse, blood pressure and respiratory rate. If there is doubt then further investigations should be performed (FAST ultrasound, CT of the abdomen or diagnostic peritoneal lavage; see Rules 52 & 53).

It is too frequent an observation that a junior clinician lays a hand on the abdomen of a polytrauma patient who has been given paralysing drugs to assist intubation and declares that the abdomen is 'soft'. Physical examination in these circumstances is only meaningful if it elicits positive signs (for example, distension or imprint pattern bruising). Do not rely on a negative physical examination in a paralysed patient.

The exceptions

If there are abdominal signs and the patient is haemodynamically unstable, then surgery is mandatory. Investigations impose a delay in management and are contraindicated.

Neurogenic shock is hypovolaemic shock until proved otherwise

The reason

Neurogenic shock describes the loss of vascular tone when the sympathetic nervous system is interrupted in a high spinal cord injury. The result is peripheral venous pooling and hypotension.

Hypovolaemic shock is much more common than neurogenic shock, and hypovolaemia may coexist with a spinal cord injury. It is much safer to assume that the shock is a result of hypovolaemia and to start fluid resuscitation while looking for the cause. If you treat neurogenic shock as hypovolaemia you are unlikely to harm the patient, but the converse is not true.

This table may help you to differentiate between hypovolaemic shock and neurogenic shock.

	Hypovolaemic shock	Neurogenic shock
Pulse rate	↑	→/↓
Pulse pressure	↓	↑
Skin	Clammy, pale, cold	Dry, flushed, warm
Systolic BP	→/↓	→/↓
Urine output	↓	↓

Additional indicators of spinal cord injury will be present in neurogenic shock, including limb weakness and reduced tone, loss of sensation or altered sensation, diaphragmatic breathing (movement of the abdomen during respiration, rather than movement of the chest wall) and priapism.

The exceptions

Once hypovolaemic shock has been excluded, specific treatments for neurogenic shock include atropine for bradycardia and vasopressors (ephedrine and phenylephrine) for low vascular tone.

Neurogenic shock should be differentiated from spinal shock, which is a temporary loss of tone and spinal reflexes below the level of the injury.

Think of the causes of PEA or your patient is for THE CHOP

The reason

Pulseless electrical activity (PEA) is one of the four primary cardiac arrest rhythms (ventricular fibrillation, pulseless ventricular tachycardia, asystole and PEA). Some causes of PEA will be more common following a traumatic than an ischaemic cardiac arrest, and these include tension pneumothorax, hypovolaemia and cardiac tamponade. However, do not forget that the other components of THE CHOP may occur in trauma: electrolyte imbalance following massive transfusion; hypothermia associated with the injury; the drugged individual causing an accident; and a pulmonary embolus following surgery and bed rest (or air embolus with blast lung injury).

T Tension pneumothorax
H Hypovolaemia
E Electrolyte imbalance

C Cardiac tamponade
H Hypothermia
O Overdose
P Pulmonary embolus

The approach to managing traumatic cardiac arrest is not the same as an ischaemic arrest: you must *think of the causes to begin and treat them if you want to win!*

A logical approach where resuscitation is attempted is as follows [46]:
• Intubate and ventilate with 100% oxygen.
• Do bilateral needle thoracocenteses or bilateral thoracostomies; the thoracostomy (hole in the chest without a drain) will identify the side of injury and direct the thoracotomy incision.
• Do FAST (see Rule 53) to identify a cardiac tamponade (requires surgical evacuation).
• Give intravenous fluids and blood while controlling the source of bleeding by emergency thoracotomy.

The exceptions

The European Resuscitation Council and International Liaison Committee on Resuscitation guidelines (2005) for PEA are to start basic life support (30 : 2 compressions to ventilations) and assess the rhythm every 2 minutes, intubate and obtain intravenous access, consider treatable causes and give 1 mg adrenaline (epinephrine) (1 : 10 000) intravenously every 3–5 minutes [47].

It is very important to treat the reversible causes of PEA, but basic life support must be maintained. Therefore, check off one or two causes on each successive loop of the resuscitation.

Patients who arrive at a field hospital during conflict with basic life support in progress following traumatic cardiac arrest will be declared dead. Basic life support has been removed from first aid on the battlefield for UK military personnel. Casualties who have unresponsive hypotension (BP <70 mmHg) or who have a witnessed cardiac arrest following *penetrating* trauma will proceed to emergency thoracotomy.

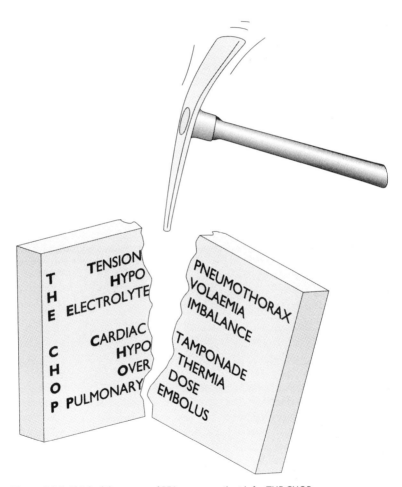

Figure 36.1 Think of the causes of PEA or your patient is for THE CHOP.

Respiratory rate is the most sensitive indicator of deterioration, but nurses record TP not TPR

The reason

The outcome from in-hospital cardiac arrest is universally poor, with as few as 5% survivors at 1 year from cardiac arrest in a non-critical care area [48]. The emphasis has now broadened from the rapid and systematic response to a cardiac arrest (*Advanced Cardiac Life Support*) to the early recognition and intervention to **prevent** cardiac arrest.

Research into in-hospital cardiac arrest prevention has identified that a change in respiratory rate is an independent predictor of avoidable cardiac arrest [49]. Although respiratory rate is the most sensitive physiological indicator of deterioration, it was recorded in less than half of patients in the 24 hours preceding an avoidable cardiac arrest while hospitalized. It is time to put the 'R' back in 'TPR' [50].

Respiratory rate is also an essential component of trauma scoring (see Rule 69). Without a recorded respiratory rate on arrival in the emergency department the probability of survival cannot be calculated, which means the hospital's performance cannot be effectively evaluated against other hospitals in the same trauma system or meaningful comparisons made between systems.

The exceptions

The introduction of a Medical Emergency Team involves a comprehensive hospital-wide awareness of the factors that herald avoidable in-hospital cardiac arrest [51]. By placing the activation criteria on the TPR chart the nurse is encouraged to count the respiratory rate as it is part of the cumulative score that triggers a clinical response at the bedside.

Table 37.1 Criteria to detect critical deterioration for patients admitted to the ward. A score of 8 or more is highly predictive of cardiac arrest and demands the Medical Emergency Team. Lesser scores can trigger a lower level response.

	4	3	2	1	0	1	2	3	4
Concern									
Chest pain		NEW	NEW						
AAA Pain		NEW							
SOB		NEW							
Pulse	<45	45–49	50–54	55–60		90–99	100–119	120–139	>139
Core temperature	<34	34.0–34.5	34.6–35.0	35.1–35.9			38.5–39.9	40.0–40.4	>40.4
Respiratory rate	<8	8–9	10–11			21–25	26–30	31–36	>36
SpO_2 (O_2)	<88	88–91	92–95		N				
SpO_2 (Air)	<85	86–89	90–93	94–96	O R				
Systolic BP (mmHg)	Is <90	90–99	100–110		R A	Rises by 20–29	Rises by 30–40	Rises by >40	
or	Falls >40	Falls by 31–40	Falls by 20–30		M N	Pulse Pressure narrows 10	Pulse pressure narrows >10		
Level of consciousness	GCS <13		GCS 13/14		A G		Confused or agitated		
Urine output	<10 mL/hour for 2 hours	<20 mL/hour for 2 hours			L E		>250 mL/hour		
K^+		<2.5	2.5–3.0				5.6–5.9	6.0–6.2	>6.2
Na^+	<120	120–125	126–129			146–147	148–152	153–160	>160
pH	<7.21	7.21–7.25	7.26–7.30	7.31–7.34		7.46–7.48	7.49–7.50	7.51–7.60	>7.60
pCO_2 changes		<3.5	3.5–3.9	4.0–4.4					
SBE	<−5.9	−4.9 to −5.8	−3.8 to −4.8	−3 to −3.7					
pO_2 changes	<9.0	9.0–9.4	9.5–9.9	10–11					
Creatinine						121–170	171–299	300–440	>440
Hb	<80	80–89	90–100						
Urea			<2	2.0–2.4		7.6–20	21–30	31–40	>40

AAA, Abdominal aortic aneurysm; GCS, Glasgow Coma Score; SBE, Base excess; SOB, Shortness of breath.

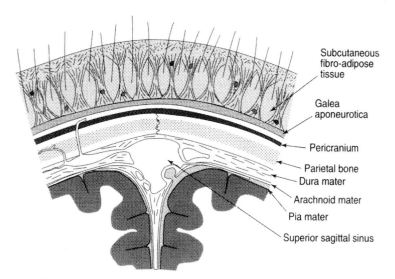

Figure 38.1 A coronal section showing the anatomical layers of the scalp and skull.

Head injury alone does not cause hypotension

The reason
The brain is contained within a rigid box and this box can only accommodate a small intracranial haemorrhage, insufficient to produce hypotension.

If there is a head injury and hypotension look for other causes of hidden bleeding (Rule 28).

The initial compensatory mechanisms for an expanding intracranial haematoma are for blood and cerebrospinal fluid (CSF) to be squeezed out of the brain. This helps to maintain a near normal intracranial pressure (ICP). However, when these compensatory mechanisms fail, a further small rise in volume can lead to a large increase in ICP.

As little as 50–100 mL of blood may overwhelm the compensatory mechanisms. At this time the brain will herniate through the *tentorium cerebelli* (where the uncus of the temporal lobe presses against the third cranial nerve nucleus in the brainstem causing ipsilateral pupil dilatation) and the *foramen magnum* (referred to as 'coning', with death following compression of the respiratory and cardiovascular centres in the brainstem).

As ICP rises a combination of *hypertension* and *bradycardia* may be seen (the Cushing reflex).

The exceptions
Infants have a small circulating blood volume and a semi-rigid box enclosing the brain. The skull may expand because fontanelles can bulge and sutures can be stretched. Infants can therefore become shocked as a result of intracranial blood loss.

The scalp has a rich blood supply and significant haemorrhage can occur from a scalp laceration in children or adults. Additionally, a haemorrhage between the galea and the skull (a cephalhaematoma) in small infants may be large enough to produce signs of hypovolaemia.

Scalp haemorrhage can be arrested rapidly by grasping the edge of the wound with two pairs of artery forceps and rolling the edge back on itself. Any injured vessel is bent back through 180°. Alternatively, use a topical haemostatic dressing such as chitosan (*HemCon*™), which is designed to arrest arterial bleeding (see Rule 14).

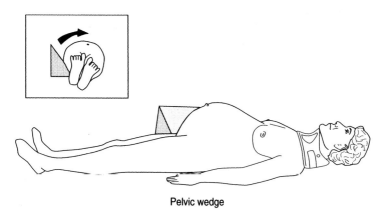

Pelvic wedge

Figure 39.1 Resuscitate the mother and the baby will look after itself.

Resuscitate the mother and the baby will look after itself

The reason

With trauma in pregnancy, the priority is to resuscitate the mother. If the mother is adequately oxygenated and perfused, then so will be the fetus.

In the supine position, the gravid uterus may compress the inferior vena cava and greatly reduce the venous return to the heart. This produces a *supine hypotension syndrome*, where both the maternal and fetal circulations are impaired. It is therefore important, as part of the resuscitation of 'circulation', to place a pelvic wedge under the **right** hip to displace the uterus from the inferior vena cava. If there is a strong suspicion of thoracolumbar spinal injury and concern about placing the wedge, then the uterus can be displaced manually.

The exceptions

Emergency delivery of the baby may still be required as soon as possible, especially if resuscitative attempts directed towards the mother are failing.

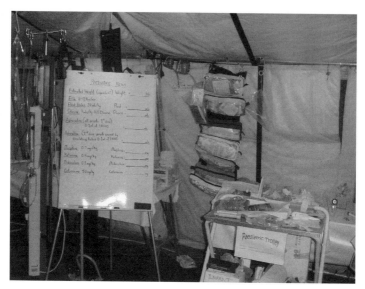

Figure 40.1 Paediatric equipment and a drug dose prompt board (the Broselow–Hinkle system is seen as colour-coded bags that relate to a specific age/length/weight of child).

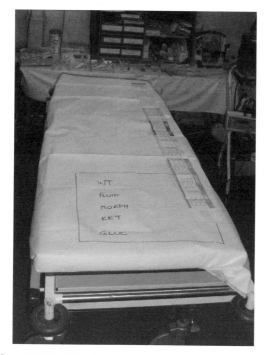

Figure 40.2 Prepare your treatment area.

Children are not small adults

The reason

There are important anatomical and physiological differences in children (for example, the epiglottis is floppy and leaf-like in a small child; the blood volume is ~80 mL/kg in children and ~70 mL/kg in adults) that mean you cannot simply use smaller versions of the same adult equipment or a proportionally reduced dose of a particular drug.

Instead, there are paediatric formulae to estimate weight, the appropriate diameter and length of an endotracheal tube and systolic blood pressure:

Weight (kg)* = [age (years) + 4] × 2
Endotracheal tube internal diameter (mm) = [age (years) ÷ 4] + 4
Systolic blood pressure = [age (years) × 2] + 80

* Accurate from age 1–10 years.

Drug doses for children are expressed in dose per kilogram. You do not have to remember all of these; normal values for children and the doses of important resuscitation drugs are contained on commercial paediatric resuscitation charts (such as the *Revised Oakley Paediatric Resuscitation Chart* [52] or the *Broselow Tape* [53]). When a child is expected and the age is known, the relevant drug doses can be pre-determined and written on a whiteboard, or the paper sheet on the trolley (Figures 40.1 & 40.2).

The exceptions

Despite the differences in anatomy and physiology, the principles of trauma resuscitation remain the same for children and adults, remembering that hypoglycaemia is commonly seen in any sick or injured child because of limited glycogen reserves:

<C> Catastrophic haemorrhage
A   Airway
B   Breathing
C   Circulation

…but **DEFG**   Don't Ever Forget Glucose!

Everyone is equal, but some are more equal than others

The reason

Within the UK National Health Service every patient who is injured and attends an emergency department will be offered treatment. The main mission of a deployed military hospital is to treat military casualties and to ensure a capacity is maintained to do this. So where is the line drawn? When *should* civilians be treated in a field hospital?

The exceptions

NATO Alliance members subscribe to an overarching policy of *universal emergency care provision*. That is, any casualty (irrespective of their background or the nature of wounding) will be offered life, limb or sight-saving treatment if they present to the military medical services.

Enemy prisoners of war are entitled to comprehensive healthcare and it is for the protection of this group that the *Geneva Convention* was created. Signatories of this convention and its Additional Protocols who are an occupying power have a further obligation to ensure provision of adequate healthcare to the occupied population.

The provision of care for children is covered within the *UN Charter on the Rights of a Child*. This charter stipulates the specific obligations to children in a conflict zone and that children are to be treated by appropriately trained personnel.

The selective treatment of an individual or faction may be militarily beneficial if this promotes improved security for the deployed forces and facilitates earlier disengagement. This is often referred to as winning *hearts and minds*. The flip side of this policy is that those who are excluded can regard the policy as an act of war.

The eligibility for treatment may change throughout the phases of a military operation; its complexity increases as the number of actors increases (such as allied nations' forces, government agencies, non-government charity organizations, media, civilian contractors and locally employed civilians).

Occasionally, the military is deployed on a purely *humanitarian mission* to provide support in an area of natural disaster. In this context, the medical care provision will be completely impartial and the mission of the military is consistent with and subordinate to the mission of the United Nations.

Civilian trauma systems that rely on personal health insurance for reimbursement of costs, such as the USA, will not offer an open access service without proof of the ability to pay (although may allocate a proportion of their work as non-fee paying).

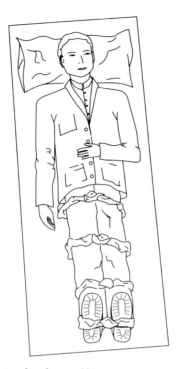

Figure 42.1 Simple splintage for a fractured femur.

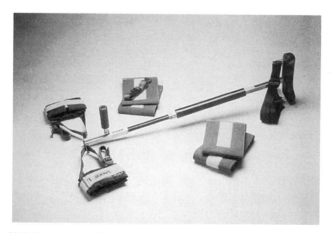

Figure 42.2 Traction splint (Sager type) for fractured femur.

Limb splintage is part of resuscitation

The reason

Limb splintage relieves pain and may reduce blood loss. Pain releases catecholamines which cause peripheral vasoconstriction, and this may further reduce the oxygen delivery to an injured periphery. Pain also produces a tachycardia that increases myocardial oxygen demand: this may be unfavourable in existing myocardial disease or after blunt myocardial trauma.

Blood loss from a fractured femur can be further reduced by a *traction splint*. The effect is mechanical by changing the shape of the swollen thigh from a sphere to an ovoid which holds less fluid. The Thomas splint (described by Thomas in 1875 [54]) was the first traction splint, and when used extensively in the First World War it reduced the mortality of an open fractured femur reportedly from 80% in 1916 to less than 8% in 1918 [55,56]. Modern traction splints (Hare splint, Donway splint) use the same principle of traction at the ankle and counter-traction at the ischial tuberosity, except the Sager splint which exerts counter-traction against the symphysis pubis.

A particularly valuable feature of the Sager splint is that it can immobilize bilateral femur fractures while still allowing the patient to fit on the ambulance cot or resuscitation trolley.

The exceptions

The desire to splint a bleeding fractured limb should not distract the clinician from his or her most important priorities: external catastrophic haemorrhage, airway and breathing first!

Traction on a supracondylar fracture of the femur may cause the distal fragment to tilt posteriorly and impinge on the popliteal vessels. Traction should be applied with caution in this circumstance.

It is important to ensure that displaced fractures and dislocated joints are anatomically realigned as soon as possible and not just splinted. Pressure and traction forces will be exerted on adjacent blood vessels, nerves and ligaments. The blood supply to the skin, for example, may be compromised and pressure necrosis can develop rapidly (common with a fracture-dislocation of the ankle; Figure 11.1).

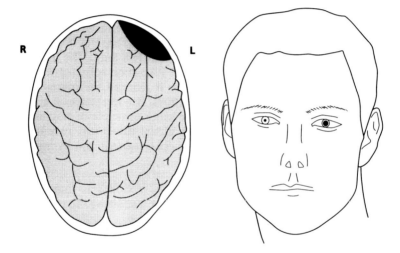

Pupil dilated same side as injury

Figure 43.1 Assessment of pupils.

The Glasgow Coma Scale does not measure prognosis

The reason

The Glasgow Coma Scale (GCS) is a measure of brain function at the time the test is performed. It is not an indicator of prognosis. The GCS is a summative assessment of the best motor, verbal and eye-opening responses, with a maximum score of 15 and a minimum score of 3. If there is a different response in opposite limbs then the best response is recorded [57].

Motor response	Verbal response	Eye opening
6 Obeys commands	5 Orientated	4 Spontaneous
5 Localizes pain	4 Confused	3 To voice
4 Withdraws from pain	3 Inappropriate words	2 To pain
3 Abnormal flexion	2 Incomprehensible sounds	1 None
2 Abnormal extension	1 None	
1 None		

In general, a GCS of <9 indicates a severe head injury, a GCS of 9–12 indicates a moderate head injury and a GCS >12 suggests a mild head injury. However, this can be misleading because the GCS can be reduced to as low as 3 in a hypoxic patient without a significant head injury, and a patient developing a potentially lethal extradural haemorrhage may be fully alert with a GCS of 15 during the 'lucid interval'. It is much more important to record the *trend* in GCS over time and to be wary of changes in the level of response. If the GCS falls by 2 points or more this is a significant deterioration.

A GCS of 8 is defined as 'coma' and indicates a threat to the patient's airway. **When the GCS is 8, proceed now to intubate!**

The neurological examination in trauma would be incomplete without an assessment of pupils and a search for lateralizing signs (unilateral weakness or altered sensation); a dilated pupil suggests an expanding intracranial haematoma on the *same side* (Figure 43.1).

The exceptions

The GCS is used as an outcome measure when incorporated into one of the physiological scoring systems, such as the *Revised Trauma Score* [58], *TRISS Methodology* [59] or *A Severity Characterization of Trauma* (ASCOT) [60].

GCS cannot be applied to small children. A paediatric version of the GCS (the *Paediatric Coma Scale*) is described [61]. An additional tool, the *CHOP Infant Coma Scale*, can be applied consistently to children <2 years old. It parallels GCS, relies on objective behavioural observations and can be used with intubated patients [62].

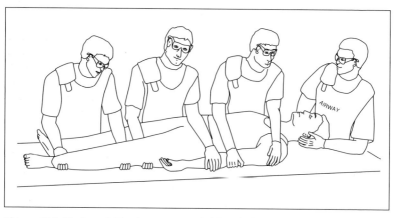

Figure 44.1 The log roll. The doctor or nurse holding the head will give the orders controlling the roll.

A patient has a front and a back, two sides, a top and a bottom *or* Roll the patient three over, three under

The reason

If injuries are not to be missed, each patient must be completely exposed and rolled in a controlled manner on to their side to look at the back (the so-called *log roll*). Missed wounds on the back can be a cause of fatal exsanguination. The index of suspicion should be particularly high with penetrating trauma. Do not assume the patient has a single frontal stab wound. If you can only see one bullet wound, are you missing the exit (or entrance) wound on the back?

To perform a log roll four people are required. The individual controlling the head and cervical spine immobilization gives the instructions. Use a command that cannot be misinterpreted, such as 'Ready...brace...roll!' Where an ambiguous command is given such as '1...2...3...roll!', then some will start to move on '3' and some will start on 'roll'.

Three other staff place their hands in the position illustrated (Figure 44.1; *three over, three under*). If there are injuries on one side, roll the patient onto the **uninjured** side. Ensure all straps are removed from the spinal board prior to rolling, to enable the spinal board to be taken away without dragging straps underneath the body. A handheld vacuum cleaner is useful to remove glass and stone pieces from the trolley while the patient is on his or her side.

The exceptions

Complete exposure has to be considered in the context of the patient's environment, which is particularly true outside hospital. Additionally, in the pre-hospital phase, time would not permit complete exposure and examination and the emphasis is on <C>ABC priorities.

Once in hospital you need to see all of the patient, but not necessarily all at the same time. Children have a larger surface area to volume ratio than adults and will cool very quickly, especially if they are wet and immobile through injury or coma. Active measures should be taken to protect the patient from hypothermia (see Rule 47).

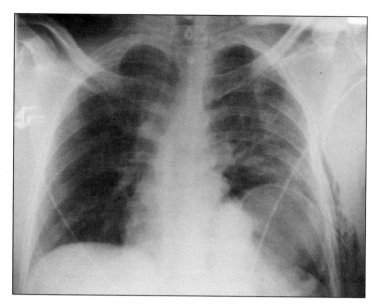

Figure 45.1 Left-sided diaphragmatic hernia. Bowel may be palpable on finger sweep during chest drain insertion.

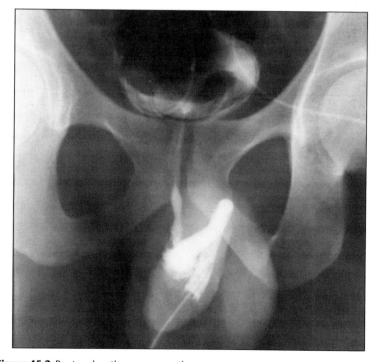

Figure 45.2 Ruptured urethra seen on urethrogram.

Put a finger in before putting a tube in

The reason

Finger before chest drain

After blunt dissection through the chest wall, a 360° finger sweep should be performed before inserting a chest drain [63]. This will exclude a pleural adhesion (in which case an alternative site for the drain should be sought) or intrathoracic abdominal contents (in which case a drain must be inserted because a pneumothorax has now been produced, but the patient is not anticipated to improve without surgery to repair the diaphragm).

Finger before urinary catheter

A rectal examination is required before inserting a urinary catheter in men to identify the possibility of urethral injury, which is suggested by a high-riding prostate. Other signs of urethral injury are perineal or scrotal bruising, an inability to pass urine and blood at the meatus. The rectal examination is also useful to exclude blood in the bowel from bowel injury and to check sphincter tone, which may be absent in spinal cord injury.

Finger before endotracheal tube

The little finger of the patient can be used as a rough guide, particularly in children, to estimate the correct internal diameter of the endotracheal tube.

The exceptions

Following urethral injury, a catheter may be passed if the integrity of the urethra has been confirmed by urethrography. A urethrogram is performed by introducing a soft catheter tip into the meatus and then injecting 15–20 mL after-soluble contrast. Any extravasation indicates a rupture, and complete rupture is suggested by a failure of contrast to enter the bladder (Figure 45.2). If urethral rupture is diagnosed, a suprapubic catheter should be passed and the opinion of a urologist sought.

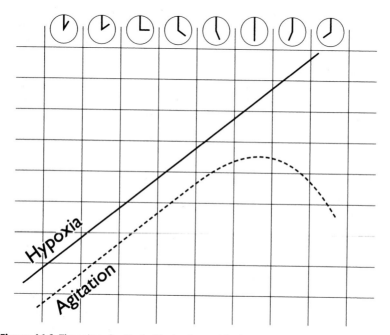

Figure 46.1 The agitated patient will calm down while deteriorating.

The agitated patient will calm down while deteriorating

The reason

Moderate hypoxia will lead to disorientation, aggression and a tendency to be abusive to the attending medical staff. If nothing is done to improve oxygenation, the patient's cerebral function will deteriorate and he or she will drift into unconsciousness. This is a pre-terminal event, but may be misinterpreted as an improvement by those struggling to control an individual who has been fighting every attempt at assessment and treatment.

It may be necessary to anaesthetize, paralyse and ventilate an agitated patient in order to secure an airway and maintain adequate respiration. Causes of agitation other than hypoxia can then be investigated in a controlled fashion.

The exceptions

Agitation is common in trauma patients, particularly as a result of anxiety and pain. It is important to reassure the patient and to explain any procedure during the resuscitation to ensure maximum cooperation.

The causes of agitation to consider in a trauma victim are as follow:
- Hypoxia (obstructed airway, chest injury, hypovolaemia)
- Cerebral irritation (cerebral oedema, intracranial haemorrhage)
- Pain
- Anxiety
- Full bladder
- Alcohol and other substance abuse

Consider concomitant heat injury as a cause of agitation in soldiers, particularly when deployed in desert conditions.

Sedating an agitated patient to allow the airway and ventilation to be controlled is acceptable, but sedation alone does not treat the cause of agitation, which must be actively sought and managed.

You are not dead until you are death warmed up

The reason

Hypothermia is a core temperature of <35°C (mild 32–35°C, moderate 30–32°C, severe <30°C). Asystole will appear at very low temperatures (18–20°C) and it may be inappropriate to pronounce death without first attempting to re-warm the body as the asystole can be reversible. Ventricular fibrillation may not respond to DC shocks until the core temperature is >30°C. Methods of **reversing** hypothermia are *passive* and *active*.

Passive	Warm blankets
	Warm-air duvet
Active	Warm intravenous fluids
	Warm intragastric, intracystic and intraperitoneal fluid lavage
	Thoracic heat cradle

Hypothermia is commonly seen in patients with major trauma (where *major trauma* is defined as an Injury Severity Score of ≥16), being found in 21% of these patients [64]. The Injury Severity Score is an anatomical scoring system that is a summative score of the most serious injuries in up to three of six body regions [65]. Hypothermia adversely affects blood coagulation and it is therefore very important to **prevent** hypothermia in the seriously injured.

- Remove wet clothing/sheets and dry the patient.
- Warm any intravenous fluids that are needed. Blood should be warmed to body temperature (a Level 1 blood warmer is much more efficient than a coil warmer); colloid and crystalloid should be stored in a warm cabinet at body temperature.
- Cover with blankets when not examining the patient or performing a procedure.
- Use an overhead heater or air-heated duvet (Bear-hugger™, Warm-Touch™).

The exceptions

Re-warming is inappropriate when there is rigor mortis or a cause of death that is clearly incompatible with resuscitation (such as decapitation).

The golden rule is golden fluid in the golden hour

The reason

A urine output of >50 mL/hour in an adult confirms adequate fluid resuscitation. If the urine output is <30 mL/hour following injury, there should be a strong suspicion of significant uncorrected hypovolaemia.

In a child, aim to achieve at least 2 mL/kg/hour of urine; <1 mL/kg/hour should be considered to represent oliguria.

In burns resuscitation it is common to use a fluid resuscitation formula:

Parkland formula (Hartmann's solution/Ringer's lactate)
Weight (kg) × % burn × 4 = mL crystalloid per 24 hours (half in first 8 hours)

Burns institutions may recommend anything from 2 to 4 mL/kg/% burn and these formulae must be regarded simply as a guide. Fluids should be adjusted according to the physiological response with the urine output as a principal guide. In children it is more accurate to use a *Burns Calculator*, which consists of tables of pre-calculated fluid requirements that are corrected for a child's relatively large surface area to volume ratio using body surface area nomograms [66].

The exceptions

A diuresis may be induced by hypothermia and may produce hypovolaemia. This 'cold diuresis' may lead to a false sense of security during the resuscitation of a hypothermic patient and is a result of decreased reabsorption of sodium and water in the kidneys [67].

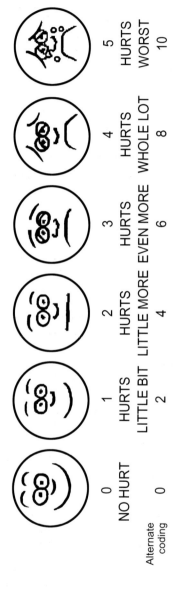

Figure 49.1 Wong–Baker FACES scale for assessment of pain in children.

It doesn't hurt to give analgesia

The reason

There is no excuse for leaving a patient in pain. Pain results in the release of catecholamines which cause peripheral and splanchnic vasoconstriction. Because hypovolaemia produces the same catecholamine response, pain will exacerbate the physiological response to hypovolaemic shock.

Pain relief can be achieved by:

- Reassurance
- Splintage
- Nitrous oxide (50 : 50 mixture with oxygen, as *Entonox*™ or *Nitronox*™)
- Opiates; for example, morphine, diamorphine (given intravenously)
- Other parenteral drugs; for example, ketamine
- Local anaesthesia; for example, femoral nerve block

Opiates should ideally be given intravenously as intramuscular absorption is unreliable when peripheral perfusion is reduced [68].

Intramuscular morphine has been the bedrock of analgesia in battlefield first aid since the Second World War. Modern formulations offer realistic alternatives for personal issue including fentanyl lollipops or skin patches, and methoxyfluorane delivered by a disposable plastic inhaler.

Ketamine is a powerful analgesic drug at 0.5–1.0 mg/kg i.v.; at 2 mg/kg it is an anaesthetic agent. Beware of hypersalivation and emergence delirium with the higher dose; muscle rigidity is also seen (this may be unwanted if, for example, the agent were to be used to assist extrication from entrapment or reduction of a shoulder dislocation). Emergence delirium can be reduced by a small concomitant dose of benzodiazepine.

A femoral nerve block can give **complete** pain relief for a mid-shaft fracture of the femur, but it is unreliable with femoral neck and supracondylar fractures.

Children may be unable to articulate their degree of pain adequately. A visual analogue scale such as the Wong–Baker FACES scale [69] will help in monitoring adequate pain relief (Figure 49.1).

The exceptions

Traditionally, it has been taught not to give opiates with a chest injury as they may depress respiration. This is unlikely if they are given in small aliquots, and ventilation may be improved by relieving the chest pain. Opiates have also been maligned in head injury as they may reduce the level of response and alter pupillary signs, so making assessment of the neurological status difficult. Again, if small aliquots are given these are not significant concerns.

Continued

Nitrous oxide is contraindicated in chest injury where pneumothorax is present or suspected; a pneumothorax may rapidly tension when the nitrous oxide diffuses into it. Nitrous oxide is also contraindicated with decompression sickness ('the bends' or caisson disease) and when the patient is unable to cooperate and self-administer the drug.

Investigation and definitive care

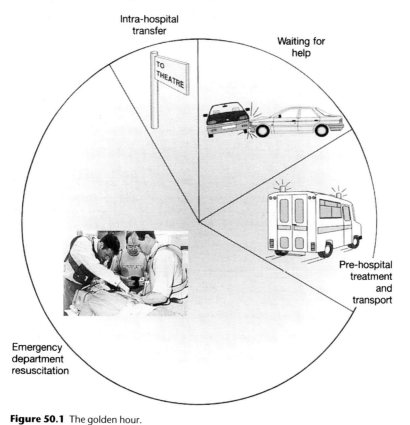

Figure 50.1 The golden hour.

The golden hour belongs to the patient

The reason

The *golden hour* is the optimal time from injury to definitive treatment in the operating theatre, which has become a cornerstone of both civilian and military trauma system configuration to minimize 'injury-to-incision' times, although disputably based on insubstantial evidence [70]. The term is probably correctly attributed to R. Adams Cowley [71], but is most commonly associated with the first peak of Trunkey's *trimodal distribution of death* described in 1983. The *golden hour* must include the time to mobilize the emergency services, to treat the patient at the scene, to transport the patient to hospital and to resuscitate within the emergency department.

The *golden hour* does not therefore belong to the emergency services at the scene, nor does the clock start on arrival at hospital—it is already ticking.

It may be appropriate to think in terms of a *platinum 10 minutes* [72] to stabilize the patient at the scene, and certainly for ambulance service personnel to ask themselves every 10 minutes the question, 'Why am I still here?'

Intervention in the *golden hour* is imperative to interrupt the vicious *trauma triad of death*: acidosis, hypothermia (see Rule 47) and coagulopathy [73]. Detection and correction of occult hypoperfusion within 24 hours (the so-called *silver day*), with the specific aim to correct an elevated serum lactate, improves outcome from major trauma by reducing rates of respiratory complications and multisystem organ failure [74].

The exceptions

In some situations the *golden hour* will slip by unavoidably. These are:

- Entrapment: for example, at a road traffic accident
- Difficult or remote environment for rescue (for example, cliffs)

In patients with penetrating trauma, the decision to operate is usually obvious. With multisystem blunt trauma it is often necessary to perform investigations before a decision to operate is made: for example, a CT scan of the brain or abdomen. These investigations will encroach on the *golden hour*.

You can assess vision with the eyes closed

The reason
Following facial injury the periorbital tissues can swell rapidly, making assessment of the eyes very difficult.

Gross optic nerve function can be assessed through a swollen lid by asking a conscious patient if the light from a pen-torch held against the lid can be seen.

The exceptions
The following cannot be assessed through a closed lid:
- Pupillary reaction to light
- Eye movements
- Structural intra-orbital injury
- Visual acuity

If the eyes are open, visual acuity should be tested in the resuscitation room, but it will not be possible to assess this formally using a Snellen chart, unless an appropriately scaled chart is placed on the ceiling above the head end of the trolley. Instead, it is acceptable to test the ability to read print on a chart or drug carton.

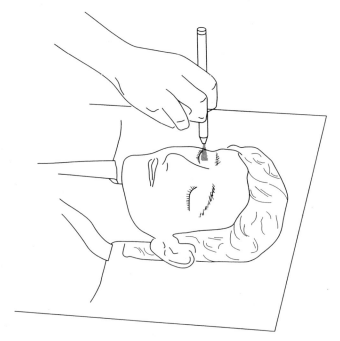

Figure 51.1 You can assess vision with the eyes closed.

You may read the newspaper, but you cannot read the DPL

The reason

It has been stated that if newsprint is legible through a test tube of fluid from a diagnostic peritoneal lavage (DPL) then the test is negative [75]. This method is unscientific and has no place in the objective assessment and management of potential intra-abdominal injury.

When performed and interpreted correctly, the diagnostic peritoneal lavage is a sensitive, although non-specific, investigation which can detect as little as 20 mL of free blood in the peritoneal cavity. It may also be used to detect perforation of the small or large bowel.

A sample of the drained effluent should be sent to the laboratory for analysis of red blood cell count, white blood cell count, alkaline phosphatase [76] (suggests occult bowel injury—see *cell count ratio* below) and Gram's stain. Arrangements for urgent processing should be made.

Finding	Interpretation	Action
$>1 \times 10^8$ rbc/L	Positive	Laparotomy
$0.5–1.0 \times 10^8$ rbc/L	Equivocal	Reassess, investigate further
$<0.5 \times 10^8$ rbc/L	Negative	Observe (chance of missed injury 1–2%)
$>5 \times 10^5$ wbc/L	Positive	Laparotomy
Bacteria or particulate matter	Equivocal	Reassess, investigate further
Faeces	Positive	Laparotomy
Alkaline phosphatase >10 U/L	Positive	Laparotomy (probable small bowel injury)

Diagnostic peritoneal lavage is a technique for detecting haemoperitoneum in the haemodynamically stable patient following blunt abdominal trauma. Its use as a triage tool in the emergency department has been largely replaced by *focused abdominal sonography in trauma* (FAST, see Rule 53); improved access to CT scanning of the abdomen and improved CT technology to reduce processing time has also encroached on the place of DPL. However, where CT and FAST is unavailable, DPL provides a fall-back diagnostic technique. It remains the investigation of choice to detect hollow viscus perforation [77,78]. In this situation a cell count ratio of ≥1 has 97% specificity and 100% sensitivity of predicting hollow viscus perforation and should indicate the requirement for laparotomy [79]:

Cell count ratio $= [WBC/RBC]_{lavage\ fluid} \div [WBC/RBC]_{peripheral\ blood}$

Continued

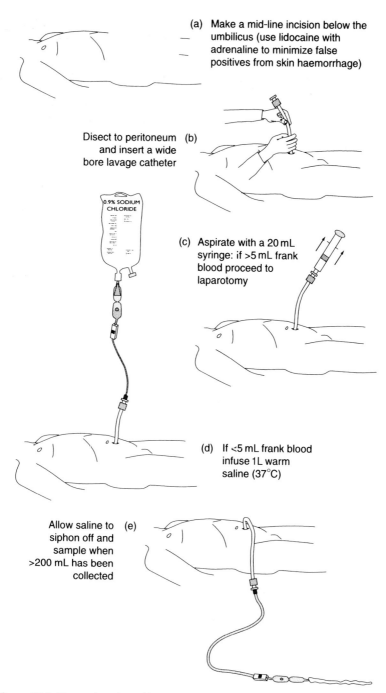

(a) Make a mid-line incision below the umbilicus (use lidocaine with adrenaline to minimize false positives from skin haemorrhage)

Disect to peritoneum (b) and insert a wide bore lavage catheter

(c) Aspirate with a 20 mL syringe: if >5 mL frank blood proceed to laparotomy

(d) If <5 mL frank blood infuse 1L warm saline (37°C)

Allow saline to (e) siphon off and sample when >200 mL has been collected

Figure 52.1 Diagnostic peritoneal lavage (DPL).

The exceptions

Aspiration of frank blood on insertion of the DPL catheter is a positive result and requires a laparotomy to be performed in an adult. As some intra-abdominal injuries in children may be managed conservatively, it is important to quantify the structural damage. A CT scan would often be preferred to a DPL in children.

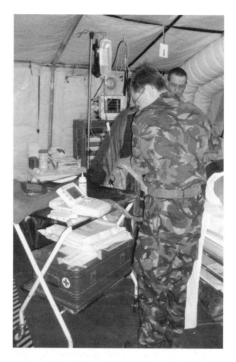

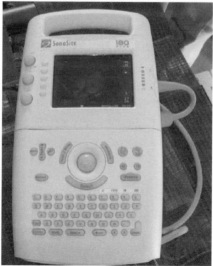

Figure 53.1 The FAST scan can be performed at the bedside in the resuscitation room using portable equipment.

FAST procedure, quick decision

The reason

Focused abdominal sonography for trauma (FAST, also referred to as *focused assessment with sonography for trauma*) is a technique that has gained rapid acceptance as a simple and reliable tool for detecting significant haemoperitoneum in the emergency department [80]. It is a skill that is now routinely applied by emergency physicians and surgeons within the Trauma Team (without reliance on a radiologist) and is encouraged within these doctors' higher professional training. There is a compensating reduction in the requirement for diagnostic peritoneal lavage (see Rule 52) or CT imaging.

The principal attraction of FAST is that it can be performed at the bedside in the resuscitation room and will immediately influence management. *Sick patients travel badly* and if moving the patient to the CT scanner can be avoided by an investigation in the resuscitation room then this will speed up the time to definitive care and limit the risk to the patient.

FAST looks for free fluid in four areas: Morrison's pouch, around the spleen, around the heart (cardiac tamponade) and in the pelvis. Experienced users can apply the technique to confirm haemothorax or pneumothorax.

The exceptions

In adults, up to 29% of abdominal injuries may be missed if blunt abdominal trauma is assessed by FAST alone and there is no associated haemoperitoneum [81]. Indicators of occult intra-abdominal injury in this group included abdominal wall contusion or abrasion, tenderness in the lower chest or upper abdomen, and haemothorax or pneumothorax. In children, FAST can miss up to 45% of injuries without associated haemoperitoneum [82].

While it has proven to be a very reliable adjunct in patient management to detect haemoperitoneum, FAST is only as reliable as the trained user.

Surgical emphysema makes FAST impossible [83].

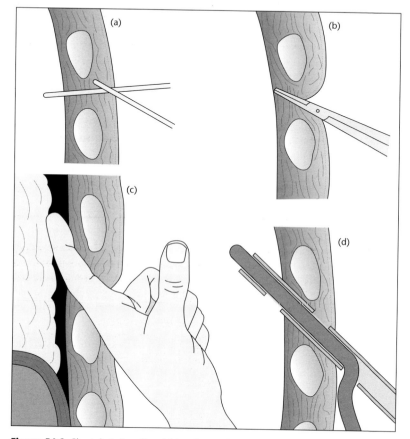

Figure 54.1 Chest drain insertion. (a) Local anaesthetic to the skin, muscle and pleura.
(b) Blunt dissection of the intercostal muscles and penetration of the parietal pleura.
(c) Exploration of the pleural cavity (glove not shown). (d) Tube (with flexible introducer,
not trocar) directed posteriorly and superiorly.

A tension pneumothorax cannot be diagnosed on a chest X-ray

The reason
A tension pneumothorax is an immediately life-threatening emergency. It is a clinical diagnosis and it is inappropriate to wait for a chest X-ray to confirm the diagnosis [84]. If you diagnose it, you must treat it—immediately!

Symptoms	Signs
Tension pneumothorax	
Respiratory distress	Increased respiratory rate
	Tachycardia and hypotension
	Cyanosis
	Hyperinflated, resonant hemi-thorax; reduced chest movement unilaterally
	Absent breath sounds
	Tracheal deviation (away from affected side)
	Distended neck veins
	Confusion, extending to coma

The treatment of tension pneumothorax is needle decompression using a large-bore cannula in the second intercostal space, mid-clavicular line. This relieves the tension, but there will still be a complete pneumothorax. A chest drain is required (Figure 54.1).

The exceptions
There are no exceptions to this rule, but it is frightening how often a chest X-ray that shows a tension pneumothorax will be seen.

A supine chest X-ray may be worse than no chest X-ray at all

The reason

A chest X-ray in the trauma resuscitation room is to look for:

- Pneumothorax
- Haemothorax
- Widened mediastinum
- Air under the diaphragm (perforated hollow viscus)

The presence of any of these will influence the immediate management of the patient, but all of them can easily be missed on a supine chest X-ray.

When possible, the patient should be sat up at the earliest opportunity for an erect chest X-ray. Following blunt trauma, a supine chest X-ray will still be performed as one of the primary survey X-rays until the spine has been cleared clinically and radiographically—but consider tilting the complete bed by 20° head up. This may help you see a haemothorax (fluid level, rather than generalized increase in density of hemi-thorax), a small pneumothorax (at the apex) and air under the diaphragm (when supine, free air will be found at the centre of the abdomen and will be missed on the chest film).

In the case of a widened mediastinum (≥8 cm at the level of the aortic knob in adults) on a supine film, which implies a possible contained aortic disruption, an erect chest X-ray could save the patient from the unnecessarily high dose of radiation of a CT scan or invasive arch aortography. Other indicators of thoracic aortic disruption on the plain chest X-ray are a pleural cap (blood at the apex), a depressed left mainstem bronchus and the trachea or oesophagus deviated to the right. Helical CT is a highly sensitive test for thoracic aorta injury [85]; wide access and a short investigation time compared with angiography make it the preferred method of investigation in many centres [86].

The exceptions

There is no reason to perform a supine chest X-ray following penetrating trauma except when there is a clinical suspicion of spinal involvement or the patient is profoundly hypotensive. Primary survey chest X-rays in these cases should be erect or semi-erect.

Investigation must never impede resuscitation

The reason

Investigations are available to:

- Clarify equivocal signs: for example, FAST scan
- Confirm clinical suspicions: for example, CT brain scan
- Plan management: for example, X-ray long bones

It is important that these investigations do not interfere with resuscitation along <C>ABC lines. If a patient clinically has an abdomen distended with blood, a laparotomy is required, not a CT scan. Equally, life-saving surgery for intra-abdominal haemorrhage takes precedence over imaging of the spine for suspected injury. The patient will die immediately from blood loss, but will not (in general) die immediately in hospital from a spinal injury.

The exceptions

Investigations are also available to rule out clinically undetected injury: for example, primary survey X-rays. The primary survey X-rays are part of the resuscitation, as the following serious injuries can easily be missed clinically:

Chest	Pneumothorax or haemothorax
	Contained aortic rupture
Pelvis	Stable pelvic fracture
Cervical spine	Fracture or dislocation

Obtaining blood for cross-match is part of the trauma resuscitation and is best performed immediately after insertion of an intravenous cannula. A blood glucose estimation (capillary test is enough initially: for example, *BM-stix*™ or *Glucostix*™) should be considered part of the resuscitation in children, as hypoglycaemia is a common sequela of childhood illness or injury.

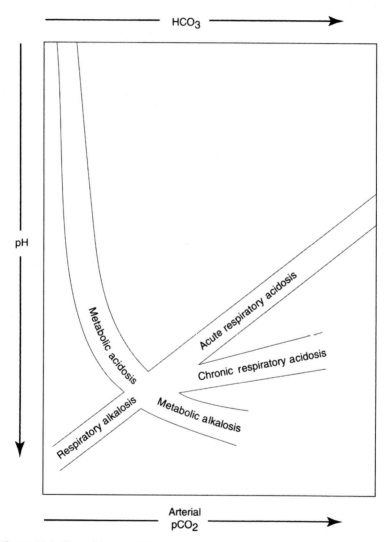

Figure 57.1 The acid–base diagram.

Serial blood gases are the signposts on the road to resuscitation

The reason

Shock is present when there is inadequate organ perfusion and tissue oxygenation, leading to anaerobic respiration and lactic acidosis. Lactic acidosis can be quantified as the base excess, which can be measured from an arterial sample of blood.

If resuscitation of a shocked patient is effective, tissue perfusion will improve, the lactate will be cleared and the base excess will move towards normal. If it is inadequate, lactate will accumulate further and the base excess will continue to deteriorate.

Serial arterial blood gas estimations should be performed on every severely injured patient in hospital, and should be repeated at regular intervals during the resuscitation.

The exceptions

If there is a clear clinical indication to pass an endotracheal tube, do not wait for blood gas results before deciding to intubate.

In trauma cardiac arrest, there is a reduced volume of CO_2 delivered to the alveoli for clearance. A *paradoxical respiratory alkalosis* can be seen when there is arterial hypocarbia, despite the persistent venous acidosis resulting from the high venous concentrations of CO_2 and lactic acid. Following cardiac arrest, a central venous sample should be used to determine the patient's pH, while an arterial sample will determine whether the patient is being adequately oxygenated [87].

Patients are transferred, not their injuries or investigations

The reason

All patients are people. If we forget this we are simply technicians, not clinicians.

So remember to say, 'This is Mr Smith. He is 40 and has a ruptured spleen', rather than, 'This is the 40-year-old ruptured spleen'.

Also, consider that relatives may be within earshot of the resuscitation room or in the resuscitation room (particularly in the case of paediatric trauma). What you say is often remembered long after the patient has been discharged (or died).

The exceptions

The expression, 'This is the kidney for theatre' may be used to refer to the donor organ!

Never believe a transferring hospital

The reason

When a patient is transferred from one hospital to another the receiving hospital must perform a complete reassessment. Injuries may have been missed by the initial hospital, or the patient may have deteriorated in transit [88]. The Trauma Team should be activated to assess an inter-hospital transfer. Do not allow a patient with multisystem trauma to go direct to the CT scanner on arrival and bypass the emergency department. In this circumstance, **the radiology department is a dangerous place**.

Sick patients transfer badly

Monitoring is less accurate when moving, and treatment is restricted. Always ensure that the airway, breathing and circulation are stable before transfer. Elective intubation should be considered if any problems with the airway or ventilation are anticipated. It is relatively easy to do this in the controlled environment of the emergency department, but very difficult to do in an ambulance (and near impossible to do in a helicopter) when the patient suddenly deteriorates. The patient must have an appropriately qualified escort. In the case of inter-hospital transfer of a seriously injured patient, this would usually be a doctor with anaesthetic and trauma resuscitation skills.

When accepting a trauma patient from another hospital, it is important to remember that the referring hospital may not deal with major trauma on a regular basis. Give helpful advice and do not be patronising. More importantly, give the referring hospital feedback so that the staff involved regard the episode positively and continue to learn.

> There are additional risks when transferring patients between hospitals in a military environment. Such transfers are often by helicopter, and this will often not be configured as a civilian 'air ambulance': patients may simply be on the floor of the helicopter on a stretcher. Helicopters may be forced to fly at night and fly tactically (low-level 'hedge-hopping' with all internal lights extinguished). The flight may be long in duration (>45 minutes) and the destination may be a hospital where English is not the first language and/ or there is a different paradigm for dealing with the seriously ill or injured.

The exceptions

If a retrieval team has gone from the receiving hospital to collect the patient, then there is a continuity of care. A rapid reassessment on arrival at the receiving hospital is still appropriate as it is difficult to examine a patient in a moving ambulance (or helicopter) and changes in the patient's condition may have been missed.

Continued

There are also inherent risks when transferring the critically ill *within* a hospital and guidelines are available to promote best practice [89]. In a 6-year significant event analysis by the Australian Incident Monitoring Study in Intensive Care [90], 39% of the reports identified equipment problems and 61% identified patient management issues including poor communication and inadequate monitoring. Serious adverse outcomes occurred in 31%.

Better a negative laparotomy than a positive postmortem

The reason

If a patient remains hypotensive despite fluid resuscitation, the possibility of undetected intra-abdominal haemorrhage should be considered. Although it is undesirable to perform an unnecessary laparotomy in patients with abdominal trauma, it is more serious to delay exploration and incur avoidable morbidity or mortality [91].

No investigation is perfect and a negative FAST, abdominal CT scan or diagnostic peritoneal lavage should not dissuade the surgeon from performing a laparotomy in a deteriorating patient.

The exceptions

Before proceeding with laparotomy for unexplained hypotension it is important to have first excluded hidden blood loss into other body compartments (see Rule 28).

Negative laparotomy is associated with an increased length of stay [92] and an increased morbidity, especially small bowel obstruction, but this risk is considered small especially when extensive operative dissection is not necessary [93].

In a study of 254 patients who underwent non-therapeutic laparotomy (where the mechanism was *penetrating* trauma in 98%), there was a significant morbidity when complications were recorded prospectively. Complications were present in 43% and included atelectasis, pneumonia, prolonged ileus and wound infection [94]. The use of laparoscopy after *penetrating* abdominal trauma is associated with a decrease in the negative laparotomy rate [95]; in addition, the morbidity and hospital stay are significantly less ($P < 0.01$) for patients with abdominal gunshot wounds who have a negative diagnostic laparoscopy versus a negative laparotomy [96].

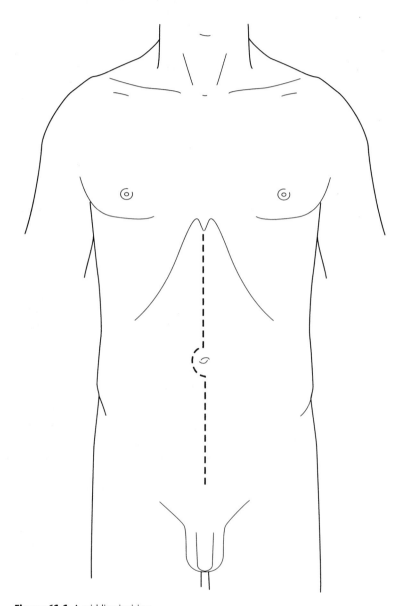

Figure 61.1 A mid-line incision.

Go down the middle and be liberal

The reason

A mid-line incision provides good access to all abdominal and pelvic structures and can be extended into the chest as a thoracotomy or median sternotomy. A laparotomy is the only intervention that will salvage a patient with exsanguinating intra-abdominal haemorrhage, and it can be performed in the operating theatre by any surgeon with basic experience. A senior surgeon should be summoned, but time should not be wasted while waiting for this surgeon to arrive.

Once the junior surgeon has opened the abdomen, free blood and clots should be rapidly evacuated and haemorrhage temporarily tamponaded. Tamponade is achieved by packing the left upper quadrant around the spleen, packing the right upper quadrant around and beneath the liver, applying a haemostat to a free bleeder in the mesentery or mesocolon and packing the pelvic cavity if a large retroperitoneal haematoma is present. Immediate efforts should not be made to identify and arrest haemorrhage. These strategies can allow time for further transfusion and the arrival of a senior colleague. The definitive control of bleeding can then proceed in a more controlled fashion.

The exceptions

When dealing with a stab wound to the abdomen of a stable patient, it is appropriate to first perform a laparoscopy through a separate sub-umbilical incision to observe if the peritoneum is breached. If it is not breached then the wound can be explored and repaired. If the peritoneum is breached then a laparotomy is required, irrespective of other laparoscopic findings.

Laparoscopic surgery is generally unavailable in deployed field hospitals. However, senior surgeons are always available so temporizing techniques by a junior surgeon to obtain haemostasis are inapplicable.

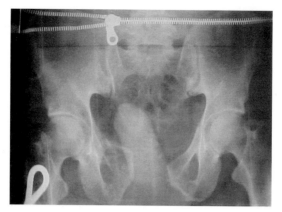

Figure 62.1 Antero-posterior fracture (an 'open book' fracture).

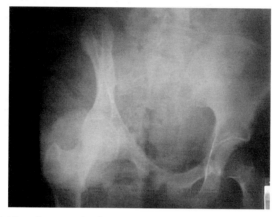

Figure 62.2 A lateral compression fracture.

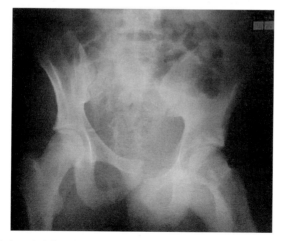

Figure 62.3 A vertical shear fracture.

Fix the pelvis to fix the bleeding

The reason

The pelvis has a rich blood supply. Major blood vessels are in intimate contact with the pelvic bones. A displaced pelvic ring fracture may result in tearing of these vessels, and specifically the iliac vessels, with resultant life-threatening haemorrhage. By reducing and fixing the fracture the bleeding may be tamponaded.

To be accurate, pelvic stabilization is particularly recommended for the group of patients who have a contained haematoma and who have sustained hypotension despite fluid resuscitation. Over 60% of patients with haemorrhage from unstable pelvic fractures will respond to fluid resuscitation alone, without the need for an external fixator, because the inherent natural boundaries of the pelvis result in spontaneous tamponade [97]. In those patients where a pelvic haematoma ruptures intraperitoneally, haemorrhage is often fatal [98].

In the resuscitation room effective pelvic stabilization can be achieved by an external splint [99]: this may be a sheet or broadly folded triangular bandages tied around the pelvis, or a commercial pelvic binding splint (for example, SAM™ or T-POD™). Military antishock trousers [100] (pneumatic antishock garment) can also be used for emergency pelvic stabilization, although these have lost popularity.

The pelvis is stabilized surgically with an external fixator. If a laparotomy is required the pelvis should be fixed before the incision, otherwise the tamponade is released without further bleeding being controlled and haemorrhage may be fatal.

The exceptions

Fixation may not be enough to stop the bleeding, and angiography with embolization may be required [101]. Angiography has been recommended as a primary intervention for some groups of patients, although the evidence is limited [102]. Despite the use of the appropriate treatment pelvic trauma mortality remains approximately 10%.

Biology is the mother of all fixation

The reason

When a bone breaks, the natural biological process is that the broken ends will unite and heal. The more surgical interference there is with a fracture, the more interference there is with bone healing. Specifically, over-rigid fixation will reduce the ability of bone to heal.

Correction of malalignment, rotation and shortening are all important for long-bone fractures, and fixation should be stable but not rigid.

The risk of infection generally precludes open reduction and internal fixation of fractures in field conditions. External fixation is a popular treatment in military environments, but there is an early failure rate when used to manage war injuries [103]. Pin tract infection is common with external fixation and antimicrobial coated pins have been advocated [104,105]. The use of skeletal traction and plaster of Paris should not be forgotten as a simple and acceptable alternative (for example, the *Tobruk splint* for a fractured femur utilized by the British Army in the Second World War—it is actually a *Thomas splint* re-enforced with plaster of Paris for additional stability during transport).

The exceptions

As near perfect and rigid immobilization as possible is recommended for intra-articular fractures and for those fractures of the adult forearm that, if inadequately treated, may interfere with pronation and supination.

The solution to pollution is dilution

The reason

The main solution to contamination (pollution) of a wound is copious irrigation (dilution) rather than antibiotics. The solution used, whether it is sterile water or normal saline, is not critical as it is not absorbed, but it should be warmed to body temperature.

The irrigating solution is best delivered directly from the end of a giving set connected to the bag of fluid. Ten litres of fluid may be used to irrigate an open long-bone fracture.

The treatment of wounds contaminated with chemical warfare agents requires special consideration. All casualties entering a medical facility following a chemical attack will be considered contaminated and will undergo standard decontamination procedures which involve the removal of clothes and washing with 0.5% hypochlorite solution. Bandages should be removed, then replaced if there is continued bleeding. Tourniquets should be replaced (decontaminating the skin under the original tourniquet) and splints thoroughly decontaminated or exchanged. New dressings that are subsequently removed in the operating theatre should be submerged in 5% hypochlorite or sealed in a plastic bag.

The potential risk to the surgeon is realistically very small, but arises from contaminated foreign bodies in the wound or the presence of thickened agents (although survival to hospital after wound contamination with a thickened agent would be unlikely). Off-gassing of vapour from a wound is considered negligible and does not demand the need for the surgeon to wear a respirator.

The exceptions

The life-threatening complications of a wound must be dealt with before a wound toilet. Dirty and non-viable tissue should be removed rather than just irrigated.

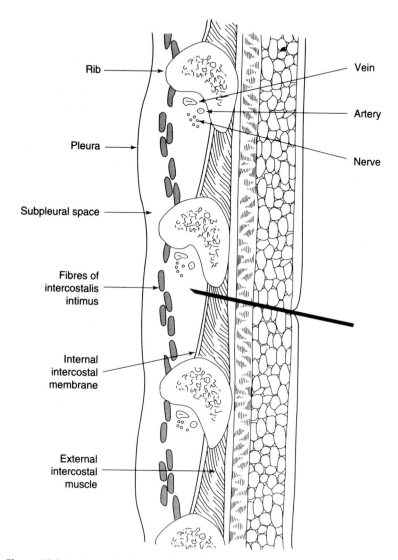

Figure 65.1 Anatomy of an intercostal nerve block. (After Nunn & Slavin [106].)

It doesn't pay to be complacent about an elderly fracture of the rib

The reason

Rib fractures are very painful, and if such an injury is sustained by an elderly patient, a heavy smoker or a patient with existing chronic bronchitis then the pain may be enough to prevent the patient from clearing secretions by coughing. Fatal pneumonia can develop rapidly.

Always consider admitting such patients for analgesia and chest physiotherapy. Analgesic options include intercostal local anaesthetic nerve blocks and patient controlled analgesia (PCA) systems.

These patients will typically deteriorate slowly over 2–3 days unless pain is relieved adequately and physiotherapy started. The aim must be to avoid intubation and intermittent positive-pressure ventilation (IPPV), with all its complications, if possible.

Remember that more ribs may be fractured than are evident on the chest X-ray.

The exceptions

Young and otherwise fit patients with no underlying pulmonary disease can be managed as outpatients with oral analgesia.

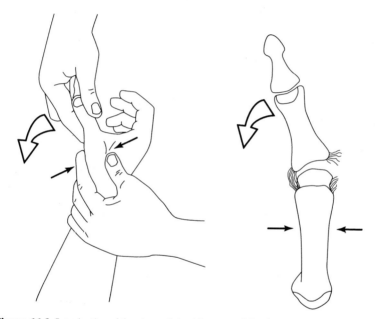

Figure 66.1 Examination of the ulna collateral ligament of the thumb. Such a 'minor' problem can be easily missed in the resuscitation room, but is potentially disabling.

A missed tertiary survey is a missed injury

The reason

The primary survey will discover catastrophic haemorrhage and additional life-threatening injuries that compromise the airway, breathing and circulation. The secondary survey will identify further injuries in each body region. Both of these surveys are performed under time pressure in the emergency department.

The *tertiary survey* is defined by the American College of Surgeons as '*a patient evaluation that identifies and catalogues all injuries after the initial resuscitation and operative intervention*' [107]. It is a repeated head-to-toe examination which will often discover minor injuries (and sometimes major injuries) missed in the emergency department [108]. This is particularly true for minor fractures or ligament injuries. Its importance is that these 'minor' orthopaedic problems can be the main cause of long-term disability.

The elderly and head-injured patients are particularly at risk for missed injuries. A mandatory tertiary survey can reduce missed injuries by up to one-third [109]. The incidence of missed injuries is higher for *blunt* than *penetrating* trauma [110]. Inadequate clinical assessment and radiograph interpretation are the most common cited reasons for missed injuries [111].

The tertiary survey can be performed in the emergency department, the intensive care unit or the ward. Current practice is to perform the examination within 24 hours of admission, and it is then repeated when the patient is awake and able to communicate. In its original description [112] the tertiary survey consists of:

- Review of the history with emphasis on the mechanism of injury
- Repeated primary and secondary surveys
- Review of all results from laboratory and diagnostic imaging
- Serial examinations
- Careful *functional* assessment of the *awake* and *cooperative* patient

The exceptions

There are no exceptions. It costs nothing to examine a patient. A missed tertiary survey is a missed injury. So look, look again . . . and look once more.

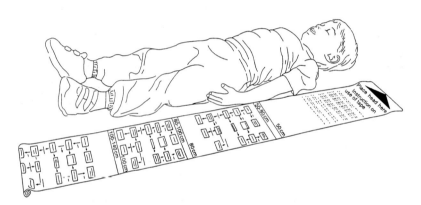

Figure 67.1 Paediatric triage tape. (From Hodgetts & Mackway-Jones. *Major Incident Medical Management and Support: the Practical Approach*, 2nd edn. London: BMJ, 2002.)

With multiple casualties do the most for the most

The reason

When you are confronted with multiple casualties you must prioritize the injured for treatment: this is *triage*. The standard triage priorities are as follows:

Immediate	Requires immediate treatment: for example, obstructed airway or tension pneumothorax
Urgent	Requires treatment within 2–4 hours: for example, compound long-bone fracture
Delayed	Can wait more than 4 hours for treatment: for example, minor cuts and sprains
Dead	

During the process of triage it will become obvious that there are some patients who will die even with the best available treatment. If medical resources are used for this casualty then others who were salvageable may also die. The decision to 'do the most for the most' then becomes important, and those who will certainly die are labelled *expectant* and are left untreated [113]. This can be a very difficult decision as it is a reversal of normal healthcare priorities.

Triage systems are most reliable when they utilize changes in physiology in response to injury. The adult systems cannot be used in children without the likelihood of unacceptable over-triage [114].

The exceptions

The *expectant* category is not invoked routinely at every multiple casualty incident, but only when the medical resources are overwhelmed.

NATO describes a major incident where the medical resources are overwhelmed as a *MASCAL*. Different countries use different colour codes and different descriptive words for triage priorities. The only system that will consistently support interoperability within a multinational force is the NATO 'T' System, where 'T' stands for 'Treatment'. T1 is equivalent to *immediate*, T2 *urgent*, T3 *delayed* and T4 *expectant*. Dead is still *dead*.

Black is beautiful, and some things are never as black as they seem

The reason

When 'dry gangrene' develops following non-freezing cold injury, the skin (often of the fingers or toes) appears black and dead. The depth of tissue necrosis in non-freezing cold is, however, often over-estimated by the inexperienced observer who may wrongly assume that necrosis of the skin implies necrosis of deep tissues. This lack of understanding has led to unnecessary and inappropriately high amputations.

Surgical débridement or amputation following non-freezing cold injury should be delayed until the level of mummification is clearly demarcated, at around 1–3 months [115].

The exceptions

'Wet gangrene' implies underlying infection. This is a surgical priority and requires immediate aggressive débridement, together with antibiotics.

Predicting survival is hit and miss with ISS and TRISS

The reason

Trauma scoring is a reproducible process that allows probability of survival following serious injury to be determined [116]. The effectiveness of the overall trauma system can be monitored (West's Potentially Avoidable Death Index [117]; Wesson's Salvageable Rate [118]) with meaningful comparisons made between hospitals within a trauma system, or between trauma systems [119].

Trauma scoring relies on coding anatomical injuries and physiological derangement to give a representation of injury severity. The *Injury Severity Score* (ISS) takes account of the three most serious injuries in up to three body regions (head and neck; face; chest; abdomen; extremity; external) [120]. An ISS of ≥16 is the formal definition of 'major trauma'. It is recognized that ISS underscores multiple injuries in the same body region (two fractured femurs is clearly more serious than one) and head injuries (an isolated head injury that causes death may not register as 'major trauma'). This limitation is partly overcome by using the *New Injury Severity Score* (NISS) which can recognize up to three injuries in the same body region [121], generates significantly different predicted mortality rates to ISS [122] and has been recommended to replace ISS as the standard measure of major trauma.

The *Revised Trauma Score* (RTS) [123] is a physiology based predictor of survival that codes and weights the first systolic blood pressure, respiratory rate and Glasgow Coma Scale on arrival at hospital. The *TRISS Methodology* combines ISS and RTS in a complex mathematical formula utilizing Naperian logarithms [124]. Any weakness of ISS is transposed into TRISS: it is, therefore, somewhat 'hit and miss' in its predictive capability, but is an internationally accepted model [125]. Death with a TRISS probability of survival (*Ps*) of >50% is declared unexpected; survival with TRISS *Ps* <50% is also unexpected. These cases require close review within the system's audit process. Peer review of all deaths is essential to ensure that results of these mathematical assumptions are realistic. An alternative to TRISS is *A Severity Characterization of Trauma* (ASCOT) [126], which is intended to overcome some of the limitations of TRISS.

The ISS utilizes a directory of injuries (the *Abbreviated Injury Scale*, AIS) which was originally designed to assist the US insurance industry in quantifying claims. While the directory is comprehensive for blunt injuries and burns, it has limitations for injuries sustained by the military, such as blast. A military version of AIS has been developed by the US army.

Continued

The exceptions

While trauma scoring has limitations it provides a foundation on which to judge trauma system effectiveness, but is only a part of the audit process of such a system. Central to being able to identify *why* a patient may be an unexpected survivor or an unexpected death is the collection of data to monitor a broad range of clinical *performance indicators*. In other words, individual aspects of patient care (such as the time to obtain a CT scan or the time to operation from arrival at hospital) must be measured if the cause of under-performance is to be recognized and the system is to be changed effectively. A significant reduction in mortality has been demonstrated within a trauma system that monitors performance indicators [127].

Stop the clot before it stops the patient

The reason

Major trauma patients are at a high risk of developing deep vein thrombosis (DVT) [128], with the potential complication of pulmonary embolism (PE). Acute massive PE carries an exceptionally high mortality [129]. An awareness of this must prompt early prophylaxis. Evidence suggests that there is an increased risk of DVT with increased age [130] and with an ageing population there is a significant need for education in prophylaxis.

Low molecular weight heparin (LMWH) is the prophylaxis of choice.

LMWH given within 24 hours of injury is a safe and effective method of thromboprophylaxis even in high-risk patients with major pelvic or acetabular fractures [131].

The exceptions

Despite thromboprophylaxis, over 10% of patients who have sustained high-energy skeletal trauma can be expected to develop DVT. In those with pelvic injuries, up to half may develop pelvic DVT [132].

While concern may be expressed about the use of anticoagulants with spinal cord injury, the risk of DVT without prophylaxis (using venography) is 81% and the risk of symptomatic DVT is 12–23% [133].

The risk of DVT in head-injured patients is poorly evaluated. Postoperative prophylaxis with LMWH does not seem to increase the risk of intracranial bleeding [134].

Death is the only certainty in life

The reason

Trauma is the biggest killer of children and adults under 40 years old in the developed world [135]. A systematic team approach to trauma will help to reduce this mortality and the morbidity from serious injury. Some people will still die despite our best efforts. This does not mean that we have failed. It does mean that we should continue to try hard to develop our trauma system and look for new ways to improve the outcome from trauma.

The exceptions

There are, unfortunately, none.

However, these rules are immortalized, and they may help you to save a life or two.

Use this space to note your own Trauma Rules.

If you wish to submit your rule(s) for inclusion in a future edition, please send them to:

Blackwell Publishing, 9600 Garsington Road, Oxford OX4 2DQ, UK

or e-mail Prof.ADMEM@rcdm.bham.ac.uk

All contributions will be appropriately acknowledged.

References

1 American College of Surgeons Committee on Trauma. *Advanced Trauma Life Support for Doctors*, 7th edn. Chicago, 2005.

2 National Association of Emergency Medical Technicians. *Pre-hospital Trauma Life Support*, 5th edn. St Louis: Mosby, 2003.

3 Champion HR, Bellamy RF, Roberts P, Leppaniemi A. A profile of combat injury. *J Trauma* 2003; **54**: S13–9.

4 Academic Department of Military Emergency Medicine. *Battlefield Advanced Trauma Life Support*. Joint Service Publication 570, 2006.

5 Khetarpal S, Steinbrunn BS, McGonigal MD, *et al.* Trauma faculty and trauma team activation: impact on trauma system function and patient outcome. *J Trauma* 1999; **47**: 576–81.

6 Deane SA, Gaudry PL, Pearson I, *et al.* The hospital trauma team: a model for trauma management. *J Trauma* 1990; **30**: 806–12.

7 Dowd MD, McAneney C, Lacher M, Ruddy RM. Maximizing the sensitivity and specificity of pediatric trauma team activation criteria. *Acad Emerg Med* 2000; **7**: 1119–25.

8 Ryan JM, Gaudry PL, McDougall PA, McGrath PJ. Implementation of a two-tier trauma response. *Injury* 1998; **29**: 677–83.

9 Simon B, Gabor R, Letourneau P. Secondary triage of the injured pediatric patient within the trauma center: support for a selective resource-sparing two-stage system. *Pediatr Emerg Care* 2004; **20**: 5–11.

10 Fung Kon Jin PH, van Olffen TB, Goslings JC, Luitse JS, Ponsen KJ. In-hospital downgrading of the trauma team: validation of the Academic Medical Center downgrading criteria. *Injury* 2006; **37**: 33–40.

11 Shatney C, Sensaki K. Trauma team activation for 'mechanism of injury' blunt trauma victims: time for a change? *J Trauma* 1994; **37**: 275–81.

12 Hoff WS, Reilly PM, Rotondo MF, DiGiacomo JC, Schwab CW. The importance of the command physician in trauma. *J Trauma* 1997; **43**: 772–7.

13 Driscoll PA, Vincent CA. Variation in trauma resuscitation and its effect on patient outcome. *Injury* 1992; **23**: 111–5.

14 Hayden SR, Thierbach A, Vilke G, *et al.* Patient turnover: arriving and interacting in the emergency department. In: Soreide E, Grande CM. *Prehospital Trauma Care*. New York: Marcel Dekker, 2001.

15 Lakstein D, Blumenfeld A, Sokolov T, *et al.* Tourniquets for haemorrhage control on the battlefield: a 4 year accumulated experience. *J Trauma* 2003; **54**: S221–5.

16 Mabry RL. Use of a hemorrhage simulator to train military medics. *Mil Med* 2005; **170**: 921–5.

17 Wenke JC, Walters TJ, Greydanus DJ, Pusateri AE, Convertino VA. Physiological evaluation of the one-handed tourniquet. *Mil Med* 2005; **170**: 776–81.

18 Alam HB, Chen Z, Jaskille A, *et al*. Application of a zeolite hemostatic agent achieves 100% survival in a lethal model of complex groin injury in Swine. *J Trauma* 2004; **56**: 974–83.

19 Brohi K. *Emergency Department Thoracotomy*. www.trauma.org

20 Mc Swain NE, Frame S. *PHTLS: Basic and Advanced Prehospital Trauma Life Support*, 5th edn. St. Louis: Mosby, 2003.

21 Greaves I, Porter KM, Ryan JM. *Trauma Care Manual*. London: Hodder Arnold, 2001.

22 Criswell JC, Parr MJA, Nolan JP. Emergency airway management in patients with cervical spine injury. *Anaesthesia* 1994; **49**: 900–3.

23 Hoffman JR, Wolfson AB, Todd K, Mower WR. Selective cervical spine radiography in blunt trauma: methodology of the National Emergency X-Radiography Utilization Study (NEXUS). *Ann Emerg Med* 1998; **32**: 461–9.

24 Scaletta TA, Schaider JJ. *Emergent Management of Trauma*, 2nd edn. Boston: McGraw-Hill, 2001.

25 Cameron P, Yates D. Trauma overview. In: Cameron P, Jelinek G, Kelly AM, *et al*. *Textbook of Adult Emergency Medicine*, 2nd edn. Edinburgh: Churchill Livingstone, 2004.

26 American College of Surgeons Committee on Trauma. *Advanced Trauma Life Support for Doctors: Student Course Manual*, 7th edn. Chicago: American College of Surgeons, 2005.

27 Watson D. The upper airway. In: Driscoll P, Skinner D. *ABC of Major Trauma*, 4th edn. London: BMJ, 2005.

28 Hockberger RS, Kirshenbaum K, Doris P, *et al*. Spinal injuries. In: Rosen P, Barkin R. *Emergency Medicine: Concepts and Clinical Practice*, 5th edn. St Louis: Mosby, 2002.

29 Cameron P. Trauma. In: Cameron P, Jelinek G, Kelly AM, *et al*. *Textbook of Adult Emergency Medicine*, 2nd edn. London: Churchill Livingstone, 2004.

30 Macken L, Manning R. Facial trauma. In: Cameron P, Jelinek G, Kelly AM, *et al*. *Textbook of Adult Emergency Medicine*, 2nd edn. Edinburgh: Churchill Livingstone, 2004.

31 Storer DL. Blood and blood component therapy. In: Rosen P, Barkin R. *Emergency Medicine: Concepts and Clinical Practice*, 5th edn. St Louis: Mosby, 2002.

32 Ponchel C. Assessment of transfusion requirements: a way to improve perioperative management of blood products. *Trop Med* 2005; **65**: 189–94.

33 Hai SA. Permissive hypotensive resuscitation: an evolving concept in trauma. *J Pak Med Assoc* 2004; **54**: 434–6.

34 Greaves I, Porter KM, Revell MP. Fluid resuscitation in pre-hospital trauma care: a consensus view. *J R Coll Surg Edinb* 2002; **47**: 451–7.

35 Turner J, Nicholl J, Webber L, *et al*. A randomized controlled trial of pre-hospital intravenous fluid replacement therapy in serious trauma. *NHS R&D HTA Programme* 2000; **4**: 1–57.

36 Alderson P, Schierhout G, Roberts I, Bunn F. Colloids versus crystalloids for fluid resuscitation in critically ill patients. *Cochrane Database of Systematic Reviews* 2000; **2**: CD000567.

37 Bickell WH, Wall MJ Jr, Pepe PE, *et al*. Immediate vs delayed fluid resuscitation for hypotensive patients with penetrating torso injuries. *N Engl J Med* 1994; **331**: 1105–9.

38 Molyneux EM, Maitland K. Intravenous fluids: getting the balance right. *N Engl J Med* 2005; **353**: 941–4.

39 Tsokos GC, Atkins JL. *Combat Medicine: Basic and Clinical Research in Military, Trauma and Emergency Medicine*. New Jersey: Humana Press, 2003.

40 Tisherman SA. Regardless of origin, uncontrolled haemorrhage is uncontrolled haemorrhage. *Crit Care Med* 2000; **28**: 892–4.

41 Rhee P, Koustova E, Alam HB. Searching for optimal resuscitation method recommendations for initial fluid resuscitation of combat casualties. *J Trauma* 2003; **54** (Suppl): S52–62.

42 Barnes A. Transfusions of universal donor and uncrossmatched blood. *Bibl Haematol* 1980; **46**: 132.

43 Lefebre J, McLellan BA, Coovadia AS. Seven years experience with group O unmatched red blood cells in a regional trauma unit. *Ann Emerg Med* 1987; **16**: 1344–9.

44 Moore BE, Marx JA. Penetrating abdominal wounds: rationale for exploratory laparotomy. *JAMA* 1985; **253**: 2705–8.

45 Ferrera PC. Blunt abdominal trauma. In: Ferrera PC, Colucciello SA, Verdile V, Marx A, eds. *Trauma Management: an Emergency Medicine Approach*. St Louis: Mosby, 2001.

46 Brohi K. *Emergency Department Thoracotomy*. www.trauma.org

47 Nolan JP, Deakin CD, Soar J, Bottinger BW, Smith G; European Resuscitaion Council. ERC Guidelines for Resuscitation 2005. Section 4. Adult advanced life support. *Resuscitation* 2005; **67** (Suppl 1): S39–86.

48 Hodgetts T, Kenward G, Vlackonikolis I, *et al*. Incidence, location and reasons for avoidable cardiac arrest in a district general hospital. *Resuscitation* 2002; **54**: 115–23.

49 Hodgetts T, Kenward G, Vlackonikolis I, Payne S, Castle N. The identification of risk factors for cardiac arrest and formulation of activation criteria to alert a medical emergency team. *Resuscitation* 2002; **54**: 125–31.

50 Kenward G, Hodgetts T, Castle N. Time to put the R back in TPR. *Nurs Times* 2001; **97**: 32–3.

51 Kenward G, Castle N, Hodgetts T, Shaikh L. Evaluation of a medical emergency team one year after implementation. *Resuscitation* 2004; **61**: 257–63.

52 Oakley P, Phillips B, Molyneux E, Mackway-Jones K. Paediatric resuscitation: updated standard reference chart. *Br Med J* 1993; **306**: 1613.

53 American Heart Association. *Broselow–Hinkle Paediatric System*, 2nd edn. Armstrong Medical Industries, 2002.

54 Thomas HO. *Diseases of the hip, knee and ankle joints, with their deformities, treated by a new and efficient method*. Liverpool: T. Dobb & Co, 1875.

55 Thomas HO. www.surgical-tutor.org.uk/surgeons/owen_thomas.htm

56 Henry BJ, Vrahas MS. The Thomas splint: questionable boast of an indispensable tool. *Am J Orthop* 1996; **25**: 602–4.

57 Teasedale G, Jennett B. The Glasgow Coma Scale. *Lancet* 1974; **ii**: 81–3.

58 Champion HR, Sacco WJ, Copes WS, *et al*. A revision of the Trauma Score. *J Trauma* 1989; **29**: 623–9.

59 Champion HR, Sacco WJ, Carnazzo AJ, Copes W, Fouty WJ. Trauma score. *Crit Care Med* 1981; **9**: 672–6.

60 Champion HR, Copes WS, Sacco WJ, *et al*. A new characterization of injury severity. *J Trauma* 1989; **30**: 539–46.

61 Reilly P, Simpson DA, Sprod R, Thomas L. Assessing the conscious level in infants and young children: a paediatric version of the Glasgow Coma Scale. *Childs Nerv Syst* 1988; **4**: 30–3.

62 Durham S, Clancy RR, Leuthard E, *et al*. CHOP Infant Coma Scale ('Infant Face Scale'): a novel coma scale for children less than two years of age. *J Neurotrauma* 2000; **17**: 729–37.

63 Sugrue M. Chest drain insertion. *Prehosp Immed Care* 2000; **4**: 85.
64 Gunning K, Sugrue M, Sloane D, Deane SA. Hypothermia and severe trauma. *Aust N Z J Surg* 1995; **65**: 80–2.
65 Baker SP, O'Neill B, Haddon W Jr, Long WB. The Injury Severity Score: a method for describing patients with multiple injuries and evaluating emergency care. *J Trauma* 1974; **14**: 187–96.
66 Milner S, Hodgetts T, Rylah A. The Burns Calculator: a simple proposed guide for fluid replacement. *Lancet* 1993; **342**: 1089–91.
67 Fischer R, Souba W, Ford E, *et al.* Temperature-associated injuries and syndromes. In: Feliciano DV, Moore E, Mattox K, *et al. Trauma*, 4th edn. Connecticut: Appleton and Lange, 2001.
68 Driscoll PA, Skinner DV. Initial assessment and management of the trauma patient. In: Driscoll PA, Skinner DV. *Trauma Care: Beyond the Resuscitation Room*. London: BMJ, 1998.
69 Wong D, Baker C. Pain in children: comparison of assessment scales. *Pediatr Nurs* 1988; **14**: 9–17.
70 Lerner E, Moscati RM. The golden hour: scientific fact or medical 'urban legend'? *Acad Emerg Med* 2001; **8**: 758–60.
71 Cowley RA. The resuscitation and stabilization of major multiple trauma patients in a trauma center environment. *Clin Med* 1976; **83**: 14–22.
72 Hodgetts T, Smith J. Essential role of prehospital care in the optimal outcome from major trauma. *Emerg Med* 2000; **12**: 103.
73 Mikhail J. The trauma triad of death: hypothermia, acidosis and coagulopathy. *AACN Clin Issues* 1999; **10**: 84–94.
74 Blow O, Magliore L, Claridge JA, Butler K, Young JS. The golden hour and the silver day: detection and correction of occult hypoperfusion within 24 hours improves outcome from major trauma. *J Trauma* 1999; **47**: 964.
75 Scaletta TA, Schaider JJ. *Emergent Management of Trauma*, 2nd edn. Boston: McGraw-Hill, 2001.
76 Jaffin J, Ochsner MG, Cole FJ, *et al.* Alkaline phosphatase levels in diagnostic peritoneal lavage fluid as a predictor of hollow visceral injury. *J Trauma* 1993; **34**: 829–33.
77 Liu M, Lee CH, P'eng FK. Prospective comparison of diagnostic peritoneal lavage, computed tomographic scanning, and ultrasonography for the diagnosis of blunt abdominal trauma. *J Trauma* 1993; **35**: 267–70.
78 Meyer D, Thal ER, Weigelt JA, Redman HC. Evaluation of computed tomography and diagnostic peritoneal lavage in blunt abdominal trauma. *J Trauma* 1989; **29**: 1168–72.
79 Fang J-F, Chen RJ, Lin BC. Cell count ratio: new criterion of diagnostic peritoneal lavage for detection of hollow organ perforation. *J Trauma* 1998; **45**: 540–4.
80 Boulanger BR, Brenneman FD, McLellan BA, *et al.* A prospective study of emergent abdominal sonography after blunt trauma. *J Trauma* 1995; **39**: 325–30.
81 Chiu W, Cushing BM, Rodriguez A, *et al.* Abdominal injuries without haemoperitoneum: a potential limitation of focused abdominal sonography for trauma (FAST). *J Trauma* 1997; **42**: 617–25.
82 Coley B, Mutabagani KH, Martin LC, *et al.* Focused abdominal sonography for trauma (FAST) in children with blunt abdominal trauma. *J Trauma* 2000; **48**: 902–6.
83 Bester L, Johansson K, Kolkman K, *et al. Manual of Ultrasound in Trauma*. Trauma Department, Liverpool Hospital, New South Wales, Australia, 2000.

84 Hyde JAJ, Shetty A, Graham T, *et al.* Pulmonary trauma and chest injuries. In: Driscoll PA, Skinner DV. *Trauma Care: Beyond the Resuscitation Room.* London: BMJ, 1998.

85 Gavant ML, Menke PG, Fabian T, *et al.* Blunt trauma aortic rupture: detection with helical CT of the chest. *Radiology* 1995; **197**: 125–33.

86 Novelline R, Rhea JT, Rao PM, Stuk JL. Helical CT in emergency radiology. *Radiology* 1999; **213**: 321–39.

87 Advanced Life Support Group. *Advanced Cardiac Life Support.* London: BMJ Publishing, 2005.

88 Dunn LT. Secondary insults during the inter-hospital transfer of head-injured patients: an audit of transfers in the Mersey Region. *Injury* 1997; **28**: 427–31.

89 Warren J, Fromm RE Jr, Orr RA, *et al.* Guidelines for the inter- and intrahospital transport of critically ill patients. *Crit Care Med* 2004; **32**: 256–62.

90 Beckmann U, Gillies DM, Berenholtz SM, Wu AW, Pronovost P. Incidents relating to the intra-hospital transfer of critically ill patients. *Intensive Care Med* 2004; **30**: 1579–85.

91 Petersen SR, Sheldon GF. Morbidity of a negative finding at laparotomy in abdominal trauma. *Surg Gynecol Obstet* 1979; **148**: 23–6.

92 Renz B, Feliciano DV. The length of hospital stay after an unnecessary laparotomy for trauma: a prospective study. *J Trauma* 1996; **40**: 187–90.

93 Weigelt JA, Kingman RG. Complications of negative laparotomy for trauma. *Am J Surg* 1988; **156**: 544–7.

94 Renz B. Unnecessary laparotomies for trauma: a prospective study of morbidity. *J Trauma* 1995; **38**: 350–6.

95 Simon R, Rabin J, Kuhls D. Impact of increased use of laparoscopy on negative laparotomy rates after penetrating trauma. *J Trauma* 2002; **53**: 297–302.

96 Sosa J, Baker M, Puente I, *et al.* Negative laparotomy in abdominal gunshot wounds: potential impact of laparoscopy. *J Trauma* 1995; **38**: 194–7.

97 Gibbs MA, Bosse MJ. Pelvic ring fractures. In: Ferrera PC, Colucciello SA, Verdile V, Marx A, eds. *Trauma Management. An Emergency Medicine Approach.* St Louis: Mosby, 2001.

98 Mucha P, Farnell MB. Analysis of pelvic fracture management. *J Trauma* 1984; **24**: 379–86.

99 Qureshi A, McGee A, Cooper JP, Porter KM. Reduction of the posterior pelvic ring by non-invasive stabilisation. *Emerg Med J* 2005; **22**: 885–6.

100 Clarke G, Mardel S. Use of MAST to control massive bleeding from pelvic injuries. *Injury* 1993; **24**: 628–9.

101 Ben Menachem Y, Coldwell DM, Young JW, Burgess AR. Hemorrhage associated with pelvic fractures: causes, diagnosis and emergent management. *Am J Roentgenol* 1991; **157**: 1005–14.

102 Bassam D, *et al.* A protocol for the initial management of unstable pelvic fractures. *Am J Surg* 1998; **64**: 862–7.

103 Clasper JC, Phillips SL. Early failure of external fixation in the management of war injuries. *J Bone Joint Surg Br Orthopaedic Proceedings* 2005; **87-B**: 260.

104 DeJong ES, DeBerardino TM, Brooks DE, *et al.* Antimicrobial efficacy of external fixator pins coated\with lipid stabilized hydroxyapetite/chlorhexidine complex to prevent pin tract infection in a goat model. *J Trauma* 2001; **50**: 1008–14.

105 Moroni A, Heikkila J, Magyar G, *et al.* Hydroxyapatite coatings: a necessary surface treatment to avoid pin tract infection. *J Bone Joint Surg Br Orthopaedic Proceedings* 2005; **87-B**: 247–8.

106 Nunn JA, Slavin G. Posterior intercostal nerve block for pain relief after cholecystectomy: anatomical basis and efficacy. *Br J Anaesthesia* 1980; **52**: 253–60.

107 Grossman MD, Born C. Tertiary survey of the trauma patient in the intensive care unit. *Surg Clin North Am* 2000; **80**: 805–24.

108 Soundappan SV, Holland AJ, Cass DT. Role of an extended tertiary survey in detecting missed injuries in children. *J Trauma* 2004; **57**: 114–8.

109 Biffl W, Harrington DT, Cioffi WG. Implementation of a tertiary trauma survey decreases missed injuries. *J Trauma* 2003; **54**: 38–44.

110 Born CT, Ross SE, Iannacone WM, Schwab CW, DeLong WG. Delayed identification of skeletal injury in multisystem trauma: the 'missed' fracture. *J Trauma* 1989; **29**: 1643–6.

111 Buduhan G, McRitchie DI. Missed injuries in patients with multiple trauma. *J Trauma* 2000; **49**: 600–5.

112 Enderson BL, Reath DB, Meadors J, *et al*. The tertiary trauma survey: a prospective study of missed injury. *J Trauma* 1990; **30**: 666–70.

113 Hodgetts TJ, Mackway-Jones K. *Major Incident Medical Management and Support: the practical approach*, 2nd edn. London: BMJ Publishing Group, 2002.

114 Hodgetts TJ, Hall J, Maconochie I, Smart C. Paediatric triage tape. *Prehosp Immed Care* 1998; **2**: 155–9.

115 Fischer R, Souba W, Ford E, *et al*. Temperature-associated injuries and syndromes. In: Feliciano DV, Moore E, Mattok K, *et al. Trauma*, 4th edn. Connecticut: Appleton and Lange, 2001.

116 Champion HR, Sacco WJ, Carnazzo AJ, Copes W, Fouty WJ. Trauma score. *Crit Care Med* 1981; **9**: 672–6.

117 West JG. An autopsy method for evaluating trauma care. *J Trauma* 1981; **21**: 32–4.

118 Wesson DE, Williams JI, Salmi LR, *et al*. Evaluating a paediatric trauma program: effectiveness versus preventable death rate. *J Trauma* 1988; **28**: 1226–31.

119 Hollis S, Yates DW, Woodford M, Foster P. Standardized comparison of performance indicators in trauma: a new approach to case-mix variation. *J Trauma* 1995; **38**: 763–6.

120 Baker SP, O'Neill B, Haddon W Jr, Long WB. The injury severity score: a method for describing patients with multiple injuries and evaluating emergency care. *J Trauma* 1974; **14**: 187–96.

121 Osler TM, Baker S, Long W, *et al*. A modification of the Injury Severity Score that both improves accuracy and simplifies scoring. *J Trauma* 1997; **43**: 922–6.

122 Russell R, Halcomb E, Caldwell E, *et al*. Differences in mortality predictions between Injury Severity Score triplets: a significant flaw. *J Trauma* 2004; **56**: 1321–4.

123 Champion HR, Sacco WJ, Copes WS, *et al*. A revision of the trauma score. *J Trauma* 1989; **29**: 623–9.

124 Demetriades D, Chan L, Velmanos GV, *et al*. TRISS methodology: an inappropriate tool for comparing outcomes between trauma centers. *J Am Coll Surgeons* 2001; **193**: 250–4.

125 Zoltie N, de Dombal. The hit and miss of ISS and TRISS. *Br Med J* 1993; **307**: 906–9.

126 Champion HR, Copes WS, Sacco WJ, *et al*. A new characterization of injury severity. *J Trauma* 1990; **30**: 539–46.

127 Chadbunchachai W, Saranrittichai S, Sriwiwat S, *et al*. Study on performance following Key Performance Indicators for trauma care: Khon Kaen Hospital 2000. *J Med Assoc Thai* 2003; **86**: 1–7.

128 Geerts WH, Jay RM, Code KI, *et al*. A comparison of low-dose heparin with low molecular-weight heparin as prophylaxis against venous thromboembolism after major trauma. *N Engl J Med* 1996; **335**: 701–7.

129 Kucher N, Rossi E, De Rosa M, Goldhaber SZ. Massive pulmonary embolism. *Circulation* 2006; **113**: 577–82.

130 Greenfield LJ, Proctor MC, Rodriguez JL, *et al*. Post-trauma thromboembolism prophylaxis. *J Trauma* 1997; **42**: 100–3.

131 Steele N, Dodenhoff RM, Ward AJ, Morse MH. Thromboprophylaxis in pelvic and acetabular trauma surgery: the role of early treatment with low molecular-weight heparin. *J Bone Joint Surg Br* 2005; **87**: 209–12.

132 Stannard JP, Singhania AK, Lopez-Ben RR, *et al*. Deep vein thrombosis in high-energy skeletal trauma despite thromboprophylaxis. *J Bone Joint Surg Br* 2005; **87**: 965–8.

133 Audibert G, Faillot T, Verges MC, *et al*. Thromboprophylaxis in elective spinal surgery and spinal cord injury. *Ann Fr Anesth Reanim* 2005; **24**: 928–34.

134 Payen JF, Faillot T, Audibert G, *et al*. Thromboprophylaxis in neurosurgery and head trauma. *Ann Fr Anesth Reanim* 2005; **24**: 921–7.

135 Cameron P, Yates D. Trauma overview. In: Cameron P, Jelinek G, Kelly A-M, Murray L, Heyworth J, eds. *Textbook of Adult Emergency Medicine*. Edinburgh: Churchill Livingstone, 2000.

Index